The Pregnancy Companion

The Pregnancy Companion

A Faith-Filled Guide for
Your Journey to Motherhood

Jessica Wolstenholm and
Dr. Heather Rupe

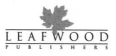

LEAFWOOD
PUBLISHERS

THE PREGNANCY COMPANION
A Faith-Filled Guide for Your Journey to Motherhood

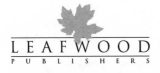

Copyright 2011 by Jessica Wolstenholm and Heather Rupe

ISBN 978-0-89112-000-1
LCCN 2010051790

Printed in the United States of America

LIBRARY OF CONGRESS CATALOGING-IN-PUBLICATION DATA
Wolstenholm, Jessica, 1976-
 The pregnancy companion : a faith-filled guide for your journey to motherhood / Jessica Wolstenholm and Heather Rupe.
     p. cm.
 Includes index.
 ISBN 978-0-89112-000-1
 1. Pregnant women--Religious life. 2. Pregnancy--Religious aspects--Christianity. 3. Pregnant women--Health and hygiene. 4. Pregnancy. I. Rupe, Heather, 1975- II. Title. III. Title: Faith-filled guide for your journey to motherhood.
 BV4529.18.W65 2011
 649'.10242--dc22

                                                                          2010051790

Published in association with the Creative Trust Literary Group, Brentwood, Tennessee.

Belly images by amyconner.com
Belly model, Angela Ward

Cover design by Jennette Munger
Interior text design by Sandy Armstrong

Leafwood Publishers | 1626 Campus Court | Abilene, Texas 79601
1-877-816-4455 toll free

For current information about all Leafwood titles, visit our Web site:
www.leafwoodpublishers.com

                   11 12 13 14 15 16 / 7 6 5 4 3 2 1

You hem me in behind and before;
you have laid your hand upon me.

—Psalm 139:5

For Hope.
I am so blessed to be your mommy. JW

For my "boys" Russ, Ryan, and Carson. HR

Contents

Acknowledgments

Thank you, Lord, the Creator of life. Your perfect love is the reason for every joy and the answer for every question, every heartache, and every fear. We pray that women will meet you in a deep and intimate way through this book. Thank you for giving us the opportunity to write it. We give it back to you. To Heidi Nobles, our amazing editor, and the whole team at Leafwood: Leonard Allen, Robyn Burwell, Duane Anderson, and Seth Shaver. And to Kathy Helmers and Meredith Smith at Creative Trust. Thank you all for believing in this project and holding our hands through the process. Thank you Angela Thomas for your valuable thoughts and meaningful insight. Thank you Amy Conner and Angela Ward for the beautiful photos. Thank you Dr. Michael DeRoche for the ultrasound pictures and all your help with this book. Thank you Adrienne Gray for your creative input.

Jessica would like to thank:
My husband Dave, whose love and support is one of the main reasons I can be a mommy and do all the other crazy stuff I do. My daughter Hope, whose life allowed me the experience to write this book. My parents, John and Janet Giglione, who have been a great example of grace-based parenting. You are playing such a large part in raising Hope. My family and friends, who are a wonderful support to me. Rex, Linda, Kris, John, Emerson, Danielle, Larry, John, Monica, Mikey, Donna Hawkins, the Stern Family, the Chownings, the Sallies, the Cowarts, the Elliotts, the Rupes, the Toths, and countless others. Jim, Dan, Jeanie, Amy, Jenny, and the rest of my "family" at Creative Trust: thank you for your friendship and support. I am honored to work with such an amazing team. Heather, thank you for taking this crazy ride with me . . . and I don't just mean this book. I would never have

made it up the mountain to motherhood if it weren't for the friend and physician I found in you.

Dr. Rupe would like to thank:

My parents—all of them—Kendall, Paul, Emily, and Lavonda for loving me and encouraging me. Russ, the most amazing dad and husband on the planet. Without your help, there is no way I would have finished this. Thanks especially to Debbie Neece and Kim Churley for their help with the common questions. Robin Carter, "lactation consultant extraordinaire," for her breastfeeding advice. Sharon Cannon, my manager/therapist, you deserve so much for putting up with me. Thanks to my church family and life group for your support and prayers. Donna Hawkins, you are my "third mom" and I so appreciate you. Thank you to those physicians who invested their time and energy in my medical education, especially Drs. Flora, Ormond, Kovasavich, Drake, Crane, and Bagheri. Also to Dawn and Priya, who helped me survive residency and challenged me to always strive to be a better doctor. Thank you to my patients for giving me the privilege of being your doctor and allowing me to serve you by helping bring life into this world. Lynn, Leigh and Kim, I'm so blessed to get to work with such amazing women and physicians. An extra thank you to my much younger partner Dr. Becky (Bell) Eia, not just for her edits but for her friendship as well. To my BFFs Bek and Wainio, thanks for always loving me and accepting me. A double thanks to Jessica for being a wonderful friend and co-author. Though you didn't actually "deliver" Carson, it feels like you did. Your and Dave's prayers and support were so essential in our adoption journey. I appreciate you so much.

Foreword

With each of my four pregnancies, I was certain of two things. First, I was supposed to do everything I possibly could to care for my body and my growing baby. Second, God was doing a supernatural work of creation inside of me. Each time, I felt so honored to be the vessel of his glorious presence and creativity. Witnessing the miracle of birth was, for me, a beautiful affirmation of everything I had always believed about God. He alone is the Creator of life. He is above all things and sovereign over all things. His ways are not our ways, neither are his thoughts our thoughts. God is love. His gifts to us are good. God is able to do immeasurably more than we can ask, imagine, or hope.

Before I had children, I knew that pregnancy would be a physical journey, but what I learned was that pregnancy is an intensely spiritual time of awakening, maturity, and faith. I guess that's why I love this book so much. Jessica and Heather have come to this message with their combined strengths and passionate hearts to give us the perfect pregnancy companion for the journey. To care for the body *and* the soul in these months is exactly as it should be.

I'm praying that, as you read through each chapter, these pages will give you direction and comfort for every question you have and all the wiggles you will feel. I'm also praying that this spiritual journey will leave you in jaw-dropping awe of our Creator. May you never forget what it feels like to carry inside your body the very presence of God as he works in the unseen to create new life. And when you hold that miracle entrusted to your care, I pray you look into your child's tiny eyes and commit every day to teach him or her about the love of God and how very good he has been.

Thank you Jessica and Heather for the obvious hours of hard work and all the prayers you have said over this book. I can't wait to give this book to all my pregnant friends. It will be like handing them pages of wisdom and peace.

Angela Thomas
mother of four, bestselling author and speaker

How to Use This Book

One morning when I (Jessica) was about seven months pregnant, I interviewed a prospective pediatrician. I was pretty sure from the start that she was "the one." It didn't take us long to connect. I felt like we'd been friends for years. She answered my questions and we chatted a bit. I'm not sure why it came up, but I mentioned that I had experienced two miscarriages along my road of infertility. She quickly offered up her own story while pointing to two beautiful children whose pictures sweetly adorned the wall: after several unsuccessful rounds of IUI (intrauterine insemination), those miracles came about by way of IVF (in vitro fertilization). I knew I liked this woman.

Later that afternoon, I casually asked a co-worker how his wife was doing. She was pregnant as well, due a few months after me. We exchanged stories and pregnancy woes and, to my surprise, he interjected about their struggle with infertility. My face must have shouted, "Me too, me too!" as I gazed back at him, amazed at just how much of a miracle it is to bring life into this world at all.

Although a struggle brings added light to the eventual triumph, I believe all life is a precious and fragile gift from God. I am constantly reminded that we cannot take it for granted that he is the Creator of life. As a child grows in our womb, God is weaving life together from the very beginning. His hand is upon us and our unborn child. But if we believe this is true, why do so many of us have a problem putting our pregnancy in his able hands?

I pray that the majority of you holding this book have had or will have completely flawless, uneventful pregnancies and births. You probably see this book as more of an informational tool—something to help you track your progress and your baby's progress. You may not jump at every cramp, twinge, and newly introduced symptom. But I could venture to guess that, whether your journey is rough or smooth, you'll likely encounter fear at some point along the way.

Perhaps you are like me—an information junkie. You just need to know, to understand. Or perhaps you are like countless others who enjoy walking through life a little bit in the dark. They believe the motto, "Ignorance is bliss." Whatever the case, the purpose of this book is to provide every expectant mother with adequate information to make wise decisions and choices during her pregnancy, while offering a depth of inspiration that allows for the most faith-filled journey possible.

I want to make something clear very early on in this book. We believe God is the giver of life. No matter where you are in your relationship with God, we hope you will realize, as we continue together on this exciting journey, that what is going on inside of you is an amazing miracle that could only be the work of his hands.

When I was pregnant, I had the privilege of being cared for by an obstetrician (OB) who is a Christian. Dr. Heather Rupe, co-author of this book, was a wonderful pregnancy companion. Dr. Rupe walked by my side every step of the way through my pregnancy. She answered every question with utmost honesty and accuracy, yet she always had the name of God in her heart and on her lips as a constant reminder to me, her patient, that he is the giver of life and the sustainer of all things. Of course, not all women have the benefit of a Christian OB, so Dr. Rupe and I are joining forces to remind you through this resource that he is the ultimate Pregnancy Companion.

We want this tool to strike a perfect balance between information and inspiration. That is why each chapter contains enough information to feed your craving for wisdom as well as a discussion of the miracle that is happening inside of you. This will hopefully help you stay focused on the One who is responsible for this life and the safety of you both.

Each chapter follows the four-week schedule of your likely OB visits. For example, you will first visit your OB between weeks six and ten. You'll see her again between weeks eleven and fifteen and so on until you deliver. By organizing the guide this way, we offer you a clear picture of what to expect at each visit and valuable information to discuss with your doctor. Some months of your pregnancy will be pretty uneventful. These chapters include plenty of extra practical information to fill that space in your mind usually reserved for endless medical questions. We wouldn't want you sitting around thinking about nothing during those weeks! There's lots of information to ponder, both medical and practical, for the next forty weeks. We'll be sure to cover it all!

Now, before we jump into all of the stats, rules, and regulations, here's what I want you to do. I want you to take a deep breath. In and out. Slowly. (This is good practice for your impending labor.) Breathe in slowly. And with that breath, I want you to take in a fresh infilling of the Spirit of God. Allow him to permeate your entire being and fill you with fresh faith, peace, and perspective.

Now breathe out. Slowly. And with that release, I want you to let go of every concern or fear you've carried up until this point and every concern or fear you might be tempted to carry over the next nine months. Let go of every question, every symptom, and every insensitive, stupid thing your friend or family member will say to you. Let it go. Let it all go.

You see, when you allow God to come and fill you with his peace, there is no longer room for your fears. Faith and fear cannot dwell in the same place. So let him in and push fear out.

Remember this exercise every time you encounter fear on this journey. You will likely encounter fear or worry or anxiety at some point. The important thing is not to give it place in your mind or your heart.

So, Who's Who?

I have never been a fan of those multi-author books that tell you who is writing before every new paragraph. So we'll take the opportunity right now to let you know how this works. Can you guess which one of us is writing this? It's me, Jessica. I'm not a doctor, so you know I won't be writing any of the medical stuff. I'm leaving that in Dr. Rupe's capable hands. Each chapter starts with medical information, and you can be sure it's coming straight from the doc. Dr. Rupe is the mother of two boys. Her oldest son Ryan is seven years old, and Carson is one year old. Dr. Rupe shares stories from her pregnancy with Ryan and how her medical knowledge affected her experiences. Her younger son Carson came to their family through the miracle of adoption.

The second part of each chapter covers Truth for the Journey, and that will be . . . yup, you guessed it, by yours truly. I am the mother of one daughter. Hope is two and a half at the writing of this book. I will share often about the long journey we traveled and the battles we fought for her precious life. We are praying and believing for baby number two right now, so you'll read very current stories about our experiences with infertility and multiple miscarriages. Anytime you wonder who's who, just refer back to this trusty little guide and you'll know. Or you can simply chant, "Dr. Rupe helps me understand my body; Jessica helps me understand my heart."

So here we go. We pray you will be encouraged every step of the way as you walk this road. This will be the most amazing, meaningful, exciting, overwhelming, scary, yet beautiful time of your life. Thanks for inviting us to join you on your journey.

A few other notes . . .

Recommendations are from the American Congress of Obstetrics and Gynecology (ACOG) as of the most recent printing of their guidelines. ACOG sets the national standard of care for obstetrics in the United States. In other words, when the book says, "We recommend . . ." the information is based on the ACOG recommendations for that topic, as interpreted by Dr. Rupe. If the advice is not derived from the ACOG, we cite our alternate source. This book should not take the place of medical advice from your doctor, and any specific questions should be addressed to her.

Throughout this book, we refer to the doctor or physician as "she," not because we are against male physicians but because Dr. Rupe is a "she" and works with several "she's," so it just comes out that way. We also acknowledge that, although the terms "doctor" and "physician" are used throughout this book, you may elect to use a midwife instead. The same information applies no matter what type of care you are receiving.

Similarly, we refer to the baby as "he" throughout this book (see, we're also giving a nod to the dudes out there). This is simply because Dr. Rupe has two sons, and she won the coin toss. The same information also applies regardless of the gender of your baby—that is, of course, except for the recommendations about circumcision. Baby stats in each chapter are approximate and may vary from one baby to another. Length given is crown to rump (head to butt) from 1–20 weeks and crown to heel from 21–40 weeks.

Last, we want to note that specific patient examples given by Dr. Rupe throughout this book have been approved for use by the patients themselves, or the details have been altered to protect patient confidentiality.

Encouragement for Single Moms-to-Be

We want this resource to be a blessing to all mommies-to-be, no matter the circumstances surrounding your pregnancy. If you are pregnant outside of marriage or perhaps—as Rebekah so vulnerably shares below—in the midst of a broken marriage, we hope that you will feel the closeness of God, your Pregnancy Companion, throughout this journey. And even though it helps to know he is walking with you, it can't hurt to have the advice and encouragement of a brave woman who's gone before you. Thank you, Rebekah, for these words of strength and hope for single moms-to-be.

Rebekah's Story

His face grew more concerned as I rattled off problem after incomprehensible problem to a near stranger: my husband's abrupt mental health breakdown, infidelity, domestic violence, impending divorce, financial devastation . . . and two children caught in the desolation. The therapist I had met only moments ago shook his head.

"Wow," he sighed.

"Oh!" I suddenly remembered. "I'm also pregnant."

On paper, I had done everything right. I had gone to college, built a career, found a good husband, started a family. And yet, here I was, my life crumbling into a twisted laundry list of unbelievable dysfunction, putting me a phone call away from becoming a guest on Jerry Springer.

Whether or not I had chosen this life, it had chosen me, as it does so many other women. "Strong" and "brave" were words people used to describe me throughout my pregnancy, words I didn't ever feel. I wasn't doing anything remarkable; I was just stumbling along through trial and error, clinging to a few crucial philosophies.

Take care of yourself. There's a reason flight attendants tell you to put on your own oxygen mask before you put on your child's. Your baby needs a healthy mama in every way, and without a partner to back you up, you have to become your own advocate. This isn't the time to play the martyr. Find whatever it is that gives you peace—therapy, exercise, support groups, church—and make the time for it. It's not a luxury. It's a necessity.

Assemble the village. It's amazing how women come together to help each other out; having your village—your group of go-to caregivers and helpers in your new life—is essential. Knowing who you can call, and for what, is the best present you can give yourself and your baby. Don't be afraid to ask for help.

Remember the dirt pit. It's easy to look at the seemingly perfect lives of others and wonder, "Why me?" But keep your life in perspective. I reminded myself that people in third world countries had been giving birth in dirt pits for centuries, yet I got to deliver my baby in a state-of-the-art hospital. Sure, my situation was tough, but somewhere out there was a single mom working two jobs. And that mom needs to remember the single mom working three jobs . . . with triplets. Someone always has it harder than you do.

Give yourself permission to laugh. A friend of mine had a stroke a few years ago, and you'll often find him joking about it, much in the same way my friends and I joke about my bizarre life events. Sure, he almost died, and I went through devastating emotional heartbreak—those can seem like things you *shouldn't* laugh about. But laughter is an amazing salve: it neutralizes the pain and the enormity of the situation . . . until, one day, you realize it doesn't affect you anymore.

Know that it's going to be okay. The day Nora was born, I was surrounded by a gaggle of women—nurses, doctors, my mom, and my close friend. It couldn't have been more unlike my son's birth a few years earlier, with low lights and soft music. This was a noisy, bright delivery room with what felt like hundreds of voices yelling encouragement —a Greek chorus of women who were telling me more than just "Push." They were telling me I could do it. I could have this baby. Never had I felt more powerful in my life—not just because delivering a baby, in any fashion, is an amazing physical achievement—but because, for the first time since my marriage broke up, I actually felt strong and brave. I heard those cheers and felt the strength emanating from that room. Then I looked down at my pink, wriggling new daughter, and I knew without question: we were going to make it.

And we did.

Rebekah Boon, 36, mother of three

Your Pregnancy at a Glance

	Baby Stats	Major Milestones		Baby Stats	Major Milestones
1	Baby is a glimmer of hope	Your cycle begins. Make sure you take prenatal vitamins for folic acid	12	Length: 2–2½ inches Weight: ½ ounce	Nausea may subside Risk of miscarriage lowers greatly
2			13	Length: 2½–3 inches Weight: ½–¾ ounce	The gender of your baby is determined by this point, but you can't find out just yet
3	Baby is made up of 100 cells that grow rapidly	Conception occurs at the start of this week	14	Length: 3–3½ inches Weight: 1 ounce	You may choose to have genetic testing around this time
4		At the end of this week, you may have a positive pregnancy test	15	Length: 3½–4 inches Weight: 1¾ ounce	Baby's major organ systems are formed
5		Call your OB to schedule your first visit	16	Length: 4–4½ inches Weight: 2¾ ounces	You may begin to feel baby movement or "flutters"
6		Baby's heartbeat might be seen on ultrasound	17	Length: 4½–4¾ inches Weight: 3½ ounces	Your belly bump is likely obvious
7		You may be feeling early pregnancy symptoms	18	Length: 5–5½ inches Weight: 5¼ ounces	Your energy may be picking up
8	Length: ½–¾ inches	Baby's arms and legs are formed and growing	19	Length: 5½–6 inches Weight: 8 ounces	Begin sleeping on your side
9	Length: ¾–1 inch	Baby is beginning to look like a human being	20	Length: 6–6½ inches Weight: 11 ounces	Your BIG ultrasound may be this week, and you may find out the gender of your baby
10	Length: 1–1½ inches	Baby's heartbeat can be heard on Doppler or ultrasound	21	Length: 10½ inches Weight: about 1 pound	Baby has assumed fetal position because he's getting longer
11	Length: 1½–2 inches	Baby's fingernails begin to appear	22	Length: 11 inches Weight: about 1 pound	Now is the time to preregister at the hospital

23	Length: 11¼ inches Weight: 1¼ pounds	Sign up for a birthing class at the hospital	32	Length: 16¾ inches Weight: about 4 pounds	Have some photographs taken of your beautiful belly
24	Length: 12 inches Weight: 1½ pounds	You will feel baby move by this point. It will feel more obvious than the early "flutters"	33	Length: 17¼ inches Weight: 4½ pounds	You may experience Braxton Hicks (practice) contractions. These are normal
25	Length: 13½ inches Weight: 1¾ pounds	If you are working, start looking into child care options	34	Length: 17¾ inches Weight: about 5 pounds	Start packing your hospital bag in preparation for labor
26	Length: 14 inches Weight: about 2 pounds	Baby has sleep/wake cycles. You may feel him more at certain times	35	Length: 18¼ inches Weight: 5¾ pounds	Do you have everything ready for baby's arrival?
27	Length: 14½ inches Weight: 2¼ pounds	Remember to do your daily kick counts	36	Length: 18½ inches Weight: 6½ pounds	Baby has likely picked a position for birth—hopefully head down
28	Length: 15 inches Weight: 2½ pound	Finish getting the nursery ready for baby	37	Length: 19 inches Weight: 7 pounds	Baby is full-term now but has a few more weeks until he's ready to arrive
29	Length: 15¼ inches Weight: 2¾ pounds	Begin interviewing and selecting your baby's pediatrician	38	Length: 19¼ inches Weight: 7¼ pounds	Try to get as much rest as possible
30	Length: 16 inches Weight: 3¼ pounds	Meet with a lactation consultant to prepare for breastfeeding	39	Length: 19½ inches Weight: 7½ pounds	You're almost there—you can make it!
31	Length: 16¼ inches Weight: 3¾ pounds	Begin thinking about your birth plan	40	Length: 20 inches Weight: 7½ pounds	Welcome baby! If you haven't gone into labor yet, hang tight. It's coming!

Note: Baby stats are approximate and may vary from one baby to another. Length given is crown to rump (head to butt) from 1–20 weeks and crown to heel from 21–40 weeks.

Sources: Gary Cunningham and Kenneth Leveno, et al., *Williams Obstetrics* (New York: McGraw Hill, 2005), 96.

P. M. Doubilet, C. B. Benson, A. S. Nadel, and S. A. Ringer, "Improved birth weight table for neonates developed from gestations dated by early ultrasonography," *Journal of Ultrasound Medicine* 16 (1997): 241.

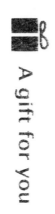

A gift for you

Hi Jillian, These books were huge helps to me. Trista

amazon Gift Receipt

Send a Thank You Note

You can learn more about your gift or start a return here too.

Scan using the Amazon app or visit
http://a.co/8LpwUgQ

The Girlfriends' Guide to Pregnancy

Order ID 108-5654586-4753801   Ordered on December 16, 2015

First Things First
Getting Pregnant

Chapter One

Key Bible Verse

Therefore, I urge you brothers, in view of God's mercy, to offer your bodies as living sacrifices, holy and pleasing to God—this is your spiritual act of worship. Do not conform any longer to the pattern of this world, but be transformed by the renewing of your mind. Then you will be able to test and approve what God's will is—his good, pleasing and perfect will.

Romans 12:1–2

So you think you *want* to have a baby? Awesome! Do you think you're *ready* to have a baby? Don't worry if the answer is no. No one can fully prepare for what pregnancy and having a baby entails, but hopefully our book will give you lots of encouraging information. If you are reading this in preparation for pregnancy, you are off to a great start. Much of baby's development occurs before you even know you are pregnant, so having your body in shape *before* conception can help with that essential, early development. Read this chapter before going to your doctor for a preconceptual visit, and you will be way ahead of most women embarking on their journey to motherhood.

Getting Your Body Ready

If you're reading this chapter and you are already pregnant (sixty percent of pregnancies are unplanned, so that's a good number of you), try to incorporate as much of this advice as soon as you can. Many of my patients complain that pregnancy books can be overwhelming. Let me assure you, no one gets it perfect all the time. This is simply meant to be a guide.

Vitamins

Folic acid! Folic acid! Folic acid! Although all women of child-bearing age should take 400 micrograms (mcg) of a folic acid supplement daily, it is especially important when you are considering pregnancy. Folic acid is an important building block for baby's development. Deficiency of folic acid at the time of conception can cause neural tube defects (abnormal development of the spine and brain). But don't let this worry you. As long as you are taking your supplement daily, your baby's spine and brain should develop just fine.

Folic acid is the most important ingredient in a prenatal vitamin. One thousand micrograms (mcg) of folic acid is recommended daily once you are pregnant. So even if you are sort of, maybe, or even just a little bit thinking of getting pregnant sometime in the next year, go ahead and start on a prenatal vitamin that includes folic acid. The nutrients won't hurt you, and they can significantly reduce the risk of birth defects like spina bifida. If someone in your family has had a baby with spina bifida, you may need to take higher doses of folic acid. That's something to talk to your doctor about on your preconceptual visit. Folic acid is one of the few nutrients that is better absorbed from supplements than food sources.

One common question of expectant mothers is, "Do I need a prescription prenatal vitamin?" The main difference between over-the-counter and prescription prenatal vitamins is the higher dose of the all-important folic acid that is included in a prescription vitamin. Prescription vitamins have 1 mg, whereas most over-the-counter prenatals have 600 mcg. Other "extras" that come with a prescription-strength prenatal vitamin are stool softeners (more on the need for these later), special coatings to help you swallow, DHA (for brain development), and a special form of iron that causes less stomach upset. It's usually easier to take the prescription prenatal because it has everything you need, and it's easier on your stomach. If it's too expensive, you can take the over-the-counter prenatal and simply add a folic acid and DHA supplement.

DHA is another important supplement that's often found in prenatal vitamins. DHA is an omega-3 fatty acid that is essential for brain, eye, and heart development. It is derived mainly from fish sources; however, most women do not get the recommended intake of 200 mg daily from food.[1] The best sources of DHA are cold-water fish, which are recommended to be limited in pregnancy due to mercury contamination. It is very important when taking DHA that you take a supplement specifically designed for pregnancy that doesn't contain mercury.

You can take too many of some vitamins (like vitamin A), so you should not add additional supplements in pregnancy without talking to your doctor first. I've heard lots of women say that their prenatal vitamins upset their stomach, so they took a few children's chewable vitamins instead. This is probably not a great idea because, as I said, you can have too many of some vitamins. A better option would be to take one chewable vitamin and an additional folic acid supplement. I realize it may be hard to take any pill at all, but if you are considering (even a little bit) getting pregnant, it's important to start this regimen as soon as you can.

Prenatal Vitamin Plan

Best: Prescription prenatal vitamin with DHA
Or: Over-the-counter prenatal, with an additional folic acid supplement (equaling a total of 1 mg or 1,000 mcg) and a DHA supplement (containing 200 mg)
At least: A daily folic acid supplement

Nutrition

There seems to be a large amount of information available about nutrition in pregnancy. With entire books, magazines, and Web sites devoted to the subject, it is easy to see how the topic can seem overwhelming. Unless you have your own dietician, shopper, and personal chef, I'm not sure how you can follow every single guideline. That's where common sense and moderation come into play.

As you prepare for pregnancy, you should cut back on your caffeine intake.[2] It is recommended to cut back to one small serving of caffeine a day while trying to conceive, as drinking more than one cup of coffee per day has been shown in some studies to reduce your fertility. After conception, limit caffeine to less than 200 mg per day (approximately twelve ounces of coffee). If you drink a lot of caffeine (i.e., you measure your daily coffee habit in pots, not cups) you may need to wean slowly or run the risk of serious withdrawal headaches. Try slowly mixing decaf with regular or switching to herbal teas. I also recommend cutting back on alcohol to one or two servings a week . . . though alcohol intake has at times been associated with conception. You may need a glass of wine or two to help make it happen.

If you are a smoker, quitting is probably the single most important thing you can do for you and your baby. Smoking during pregnancy is associated with a significantly increased risk of preterm birth, miscarriage, low birth weight, and ectopic pregnancy. Infants born to mothers who smoke are at increased risk for asthma, colic, obesity, and sudden infant death syndrome. Less is known about the effects of secondhand smoke, although it should also be avoided as much as possible. I often hear the argument, "I smoked while I was pregnant with my last baby, and he's just fine." This only means that you were lucky. Smoking during pregnancy is like gambling on the health of your child. Hopefully, that's not a chance that any of you will take.

Before you conceive or very early on in your pregnancy, it's important to assess how ready your body is for this major invasion. There are many Web sites that will help you calculate your Body Mass Index (BMI). This number is important and will tell you how prepared you are to put your body through something like pregnancy and childbirth. A lot of you are at a healthy weight, but others may be cringing right now. Some may not want to know what something called their "body mass index" is, but this calculation is important to your overall health and that of your unborn child. As painful as it might be to come face-to-face with the reality of your BMI, knowing this number and acting accordingly can make all the difference on this journey. Your BMI equals your [weight in pounds / (height in inches x height in inches)] x 703.

If, after calculating your BMI, you discover that you fall within the obese range, weight loss is recommended before planned conception. If you fall within the overweight range, you should also consider weight loss, but it's not as necessary. Obesity in pregnancy can increase the risk of complications such as gestational diabetes, high blood pressure, and the need to have a cesarean section. The more prepared your body is for this journey, the more enjoyable and healthy it will be. If you are reading this, you are already pregnant, and you know your BMI is above the healthy range, don't worry. Start as soon as you can on a healthy pregnancy diet and aim to exercise four to six days a week. Don't be afraid to take care of yourself before you have a baby. It might be the last time you get to focus on YOU.

As you prepare your body for pregnancy, you should focus on eating purposefully. Look at how many calories your body needs, and fill those calories with the most high-yield nutritious foods. There are several Web sites that will tell you the amount of calories you need for your height and activity level. The Web site www. mypyramid.gov will give you a sample food pyramid based on your caloric needs. The best strategy is to plan ahead. Focus on getting five servings of fruits and vegetables a day, with at least one of those vegetables being a dark green or leafy vegetable (sorry, pickles don't count). Drink lots of water: around eight glasses a day is ideal. Also, make sure at least half of your grains are whole grains.

There are many foods to avoid during pregnancy, including several types of fish. Shark, swordfish, king mackerel, and tilefish contain high levels of mercury. It is recommended that they be avoided even while attempting to get pregnant. Mercury is a neurotoxin that is thought to have a bad effect on the baby's brain development. Fish are also the main food source for DHA which is *good* for baby's brain development, so eating fish is healthy and important. Just focus on the fish with low levels of mercury. Please note that fish sticks and fast food fish sandwiches are in general made from low-mercury fish.

Fish Safety Chart[3]

Fish that should be avoided altogether (high levels of mercury):	tilefish, shark, swordfish, and king mackerel
Fish that should be limited to one serving per week (moderate levels of mercury):	albacore tuna, lobster, halibut, grouper, and Chilean sea bass
Fish that should be limited to two servings a week (low mercury):	salmon, pollack, catfish, shrimp, canned light tuna, sardines, trout, oysters, snapper, anchovies, and mussels

It is important for you to plan your menu each week. You aren't going to meet your nutritional guidelines by eating fast food or grabbing whatever is easily available. This is why the majority of Americans do not live a healthy lifestyle. A small amount of time invested in planning and shopping can profit huge rewards for your health and the health of your future child. Take some time to go over the sample menu plan on the previous page. Follow these menu ideas, adjusting them as needed for your family and lifestyle.

Activity

Being active is beneficial to overall health as well as health in pregnancy. The minimum activity recommendation for pregnant women is light activity for at least thirty minutes daily. If you are not currently in an exercise program, I recommend walking and swimming as the two best options during pregnancy. Why not get started now? When walking, you want to walk at a pace that causes you to breathe hard. Once you conceive, you will want to check your heart rate to make sure it's less than 150, or make sure that you can still talk while you are exercising. After giving this advice to a patient, she complained that exercising made her feel crazy. When I asked why, she explained that she would talk to herself every few minutes to make sure that her heart rate wasn't too high, and

Sample Menu Plan

Day 1	Day 2	Day 3
Breakfast: Whole grain cereal w/ skim milk Berries Scrambled egg	**Breakfast:** Sandwich with Canadian bacon, egg, cheese and whole wheat toast Milk	**Breakfast:** Whole wheat toast w/ Peanut butter Milk
Snack: Apple with peanut butter	**Snack:** Banana	**Snack:** Pita chips w/ hummus
Lunch: Salad (spinach or dark greens) Grilled chicken Mandarin oranges Yogurt with granola	**Lunch:** Vegetable beef soup Brown rice 2 chocolate chip cookies	**Lunch:** Small hamburger Orange or side salad Yogurt
Snack: Raw almonds Milk	**Snack:** 2 servings of string cheese	**Snack:** Low sugar granola bar
Dinner: Whole wheat pasta Tomato sauce Broccoli	**Dinner:** Salmon Baked sweet potato Side salad Wheat bread	**Dinner:** Chicken and broccoli stir fry Brown rice Ice cream

people would look at her funny. Perhaps the "talking" advice is best for working out with a partner. Others may just want to consider investing in a heart rate monitor.

Yoga and Pilates are also excellent for getting you in shape for pregnancy because they focus on flexibility and the core abdominal muscles. Pregnancies can often be complicated by back strain, so having strong abdominal muscles before pregnancy can be helpful to reduce the troublesome backaches. The main goal is to find something you enjoy, which will help you stick with it. Planning ahead to fit exercise into your schedule or getting a workout buddy to hold you accountable are both good strategies for making it a regular part of your routine.

Other than keeping your heart rate below 150, there is not an extensive list of restrictions for exercise in pregnancy. Activity choice is more often determined by the patient's level of comfort and prepregnancy athletic conditioning. Women who run several miles a day can usually continue during pregnancy; however, if they begin to experience severe nausea and fatigue, they may want to change to walking or yoga. They can then switch back to jogging in the second trimester, when they begin to feel better. Additionally, while the occasional woman can participate in aerobics until the bitter end, most women will find exercise too uncomfortable after thirty-five weeks.

If you are already active, you can usually continue your exercise routine while trying to conceive. An exception would be if your exercise regimen is for training purposes, or you are a professional athlete. Use some common sense here—training for a marathon and trying to conceive are not best coupled together. If your exercise is so intense that you don't have periods, then you are not ovulating and will need to decrease your activity to conceive. If you have questions about your exercise regimen, you should discuss them with your doctor.

Gingivitis

Gum disease and poor dental hygiene have been associated with preterm labor and other pregnancy complications. I would recommend addressing any dental issues before pregnancy. Make sure you floss daily and brush your teeth twice a day. Once pregnant, your dentist can perform cleanings, basic fillings, and X-rays as needed as long as a shield is placed over your belly. If more in-depth dentistry is needed, your dentist can communicate with your OB to discuss the safety of the medications that need to be used.

Preconceptual Testing

I would encourage all of you to meet with your OB for a preconceptual counseling visit. There are some definite steps that can be taken to improve your health during pregnancy and ultimately the health of your baby. If you are healthy in general, you can probably discuss these issues at your annual exam, and your doctor can draw your blood to check your immunities and start you on a prenatal vitamin. If you have any extensive medical issues, you will probably want to schedule a special visit to discuss your options and develop a plan.

Additionally, your doctor may want to check your immunity to rubella and determine whether any immunizations are needed before conception. Testing your immunity for rubella or the German measles is recommended before conception for all patients. You are protected through the MMR vaccine you likely received as a child, but the vaccine can wear off over time. Rubella is not a very severe illness for the expectant mother, but it can cross the placenta and cause major malformations in the baby during development. If you are tested before conception and are not immune, you can be given the vaccine before you try to get pregnant. The vaccine is a live virus, so we recommend waiting a month after you receive the vaccine before you attempt to conceive.

Chicken pox is another disease that can be much more severe in pregnancy. This can be near fatal for the expectant mother, and it can cause birth defects in the baby. If you remember having chicken pox, then you are immune and don't need to be tested. If you are unsure if you've had it before, then your doctor can test your immunity. If you are not immune, you can get the vaccine. Again, it is a live vaccine, so we recommend waiting a month before conception.

Genetic Disease Testing

Depending on your and your partner's ethnic backgrounds and family history, genetic testing may be recommended before conception.

Cystic fibrosis (CF) is a genetic disorder for which you can be screened before conception. Cystic fibrosis can cause significant lung and digestive problems in the baby. Both the mother and father have to be carriers of the disease to pass it to the baby. There is usually no family history of CF even when it appears, which is why many couples choose to be tested. It is more common among Caucasian couples. If you are found to be a carrier, your husband or partner will also be tested. If he is a carrier as well, you will be referred to genetic counseling. If there is a family history of CF, then extensive testing is strongly recommended.

Sickle-cell anemia is one of the most common disorders among children of African descent. If either partner is of African descent, then a sickle-cell screen is recommended. If there is a family history of any other known genetic disorder on either side, then it may be wise to have genetic counseling before conception. People of Eastern European Jewish heritage have a higher rate of carrying certain genetic disorders, so if both parents are of Ashkenazi Jewish heritage, it is especially important to have genetic counseling. There are specific screening panels that can help identify Jewish couples that are at risk of having children with genetic disorders.

Genetics can get pretty complicated. Genetic counseling involves sitting down with an expert in the field of genetics who helps estimate the risk of your baby being born with certain diseases. Genetic diseases are inherited in the DNA of the parents. There are some diseases that are always passed down from parent to child (called *autosomal dominant*). For others, both mom and dad simply have to be carriers of the genes (*autosomal recessive*). This means that even though the parents don't have the disease, the abnormal DNA is hidden in their genes. So when two carriers have a baby together, their child can have the disease even though the parents are healthy. There are other disorders that are *multifactorial*. This means they tend to run in families, and couples may have a slightly increased risk (usually two to three percent) of having a baby with the disorder. See the Appendix for a list of common genetic disorders in each category.

What you do with the information from your genetic counseling is up to you. That's where the "counseling" part comes in. If you discover that your baby might be at a slightly increased risk of heart defects (multifactorial genetics), your doctor will order special heart ultrasounds (fetal echoes) during pregnancy. If you have an autosomal recessive disorder, you may choose to have in vitro fertilization, so that the embryos can be screened for the abnormal genes. Sometimes people will choose adoption or other family planning options based on these findings. Others will continue their pregnancy plans and just be aware of the risks and watch their children closely for signs of the various disorders.

Genetic Testing Recommendation	Race
Cystic Fibrosis	Caucasian
Sickle-Cell Anemia	African American
Extensive Genetic Panel	Jewish

Review the list of genetic disorders in the Appendix, and if you know of any family member with a genetic disorder, then consider additional testing and counseling. If you are unsure of your history, it is sometimes helpful to ask grandparents about distant relatives.

Advanced Maternal Age

Technically, advanced maternal age means that you will be thirty-five at the time of delivery. Ouch! I don't like that definition, either! Though it is better than the previous term, *elderly gravida*, which was formerly used to describe pregnant women over thirty-five. The term comes from the history of genetic testing. Originally, the only test we had for Down syndrome was the amniocentesis. This test is done by inserting a needle into the amniotic fluid to determine what the fetal chromosomes look like. The test was offered to patients starting at age thirty-five because that's when the risk of the test equaled the risk of the disease. At thirty-five, your risk of having a baby with Down syndrome is 1/250 and your risk of complication from the test is also 1/250.

You still have a ninety-nine percent chance of having a genetically normal baby at the age of thirty-five. A lot of people get fixated on this age because they think that, at this point, they are "high risk." While fertility does begin to decrease with age and the risk of Down syndrome increases with age in general, there is really nothing magic about having a baby before you turn thirty-five. It's not as if at thirty-four all babies are fine and then magically at thirty-five half your babies have Down syndrome. No matter what age you are, being pregnant is very much the same, and labor still hurts like you know what! So if you fall into this "advanced maternal age" category, talk to your doctor about your concerns and consider having genetic testing to give you peace of mind. We will discuss genetic testing of the baby more in Chapter Three.

With increasing age, women also have an increased rate of twins, as well as an increased rate of preeclampsia, preterm labor, and gestational diabetes. The higher rate of complications is often related to preexisting medical conditions. Healthy, nonsmoking, nonobese women over thirty-five have only a slightly increased risk of these complications.[4]

Medical Conditions

Any chronic medical condition that requires medication, such as lupus, epilepsy, Crohn's disease, or hyperthyroidism should prompt a preconceptual counseling visit. This section focuses on a few such conditions.

Hypertension. High blood pressure is another common medical disorder that can affect pregnancy and requires special monitoring. You will need to discuss your medications with your doctor to ensure you are taking ones that are safe during pregnancy. Additionally, patients with hypertension can be more prone to preeclampsia, a condition which results in further elevation in blood pressure toward the end of pregnancy. Sometimes preeclampsia can lead to premature birth, so be sure to discuss your high blood pressure with your doctor early on in pregnancy.

Preeclampsia

Preeclampsia is a serious complication of pregnancy that involves elevated blood pressure and impaired kidney function. It goes away after delivering the baby. Learn more about this condition in Chapter Ten.

Diabetes. Diabetes is an illness that can greatly affect your pregnancy. Several of the medicines taken for diabetes can be harmful in pregnancy, so talk to your doctor about which ones you can continue. In addition, having excellent control of your sugars before conception can improve your pregnancy outcome. Diabetics can be at risk for preeclampsia, and their baby's growth can also be affected, so diabetic pregnancies are often co-managed with a high-risk specialist.

Gastric bypass. Obese women who lose weight have improved fertility, no matter the reason for the weight loss. Women with gastric bypass procedures are encouraged to wait until they have reached a weight plateau before attempting conception, as rapid weight loss during pregnancy holds the potential for harm. There are several different types of weight-loss surgeries. Depending on the type of surgery the patient had, she may be at increased risk for malabsorption during pregnancy and may need additional supplementation of iron, calcium, or B vitamins. It's best to meet with your weight-loss surgeon in addition to your OB before conception. Having weight-loss surgery has not been shown to increase complications in pregnancy, whereas obesity increases the risk for preeclampsia, diabetes, and cesarean section.

Depression. Depression affects ten percent of women of childbearing age. If you are on medication for depression, you will want to discuss the safety of taking the specific medication during pregnancy versus the risk of discontinuation. If you discover you are pregnant while taking antidepressants, talk to your doctor before you discontinue them, as some can have serious withdrawal symptoms.

Getting Pregnant

One of my favorite questions is, "How do I get pregnant?" This question usually comes from a professional woman holding three pregnancy books, two day planners, and a cell phone. I grin, take a deep breath, and try not to respond with the myriad smarmy answers that come to mind. ("Try the back seat of a car; it has been working for years!") I usually reply, "Have sex!" I know this is a bit of a smart reply, but sometimes I can't help myself. The simple answer is: go off contraception for a couple months and see what happens. I don't recommend taking your temperature or doing ovulation kits initially. You shouldn't overthink it. Just have fun for at least six months. Do track your cycles on a calendar, noting the first day and how long they last.

If you're not pregnant after six months, you should start timing things a little more. First, look at your periods. They should be pretty regular. The time span from the first day of one period to the first day of the next should be twenty-two to thirty-three days. If your periods are further apart than this, or closer together, you are probably not ovulating regularly and should make an appointment to consult your doctor.

FDLMP

Your due date will be determined by the first day of your last menstrual period (FDLMP). So make sure you keep track of this day each month as you try to conceive. Once you are pregnant, the counting of gestational weeks will begin at the FDLMP. The easy way to calculate your due date is to subtract three from the month and add seven to the day. For example, if the FDLMP was 10/10/2011, then your due date would be 7/17/2012.

Ovulation normally occurs fourteen days before you start your period. So you have to work backward. Look at when your period started last month, and try to guesstimate when it's going to start this month. Then count back fourteen days. This is the approximate date of ovulation. Have sex during the four days before and the four days after this date. Do not have sex more than once a day, as having sex more than once a day dilutes the semen. Many women want to know *exactly* when they ovulate. This can be accomplished by measuring and charting your morning temperature or by taking a daily ovulation kit. Ovulation kits are best done at the same time every day. A positive result means ovulation will occur in the next 14–25 hours. Sperm can live for up to 72 hours, so having sex daily during the time of ovulation should cover it. If your ovulation kit does not show ovulation, then you should follow up with your doctor. If the tests show ovulation, then you should continue trying for an additional six months. If you are not pregnant after an additional six months, you should seek medical attention. Ninety percent of couples who are going to conceive spontaneously will do so in one year.[5]

When to seek medical attention for infertility after six months:

- Over thirty-seven years old (some organizations say thirty-two)
- Irregular periods
- History of endometriosis
- History of polycystic ovary syndrome (PCOS)
- History of tubal pregnancy or pelvic surgery
- History of pelvic inflammatory disease
- No ovulation on ovulation predictor kit

When You Struggle with Infertility

The initial workup for infertility involves making sure everybody's parts are working. First, your partner should have an analysis performed of his sperm. Yes, the man has the easy part . . . which seems to be a theme with all things related to making and having a baby. This will confirm that he has a normal number of sperm with good movement and shape. Next, you will need a blood test to check various hormone levels to see if you are ovulating and have an adequate reserve of eggs in your ovaries.

A test called an HSG (hysterosalpingogram) is also recommended. The HSG is an X-ray where dye is inserted through the cervix into the uterus to confirm that the inside of the uterus has a normal shape. It also reveals whether your tubes are open. How will your doctor get to the cervix? You guessed it: just like a Pap smear. So, basically, you will get a really long Pap smear in the radiology department. Not completely fun, but at least the hospital will ensure your privacy and make sure it doesn't take very long. Many women say that the test makes them feel crampy, so take some ibuprofen before the procedure. The great thing about an HSG is that simply having the test done can improve your fertility. Some think the test can be curative. For example, if there is a bit of mucus stuck in one of your tubes, the test can flush it out, helping to open the tube. Based on the results of this test, your doctor will advise you on the next steps to take to conceive.

Many couples are concerned about fertility treatments and testing. They tell me they don't want seven babies at once! There are usually very simple things that can be done to improve fertility, and you shouldn't be pressured into doing *any* aggressive treatments or tests if you do not feel comfortable with them. Talk through your options with your doctor and then discuss them with your spouse or partner to determine the course of action you want to take.

His and Hers Initial Infertility Workup

His	Hers
Physical exam	Physical exam
Semen analysis	Ultrasound
	Hormone levels
	HSG

About twenty-five percent of the time, everything turns out normal with the testing, and no problems are found. This is called *unexplained infertility* and is actually not great news. From a medical standpoint, it's better to find something that we can fix, rather than infertility from an unknown cause. If this is true in your case, you may want to seek additional testing from an infertility specialist.

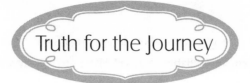

Truth for the Journey

Therefore, I urge you brothers, in view of God's mercy, to offer your bodies as living sacrifices, holy and pleasing to God—this is your spiritual act of worship. Do not conform any longer to the pattern of this world, but be transformed by the renewing of your mind. Then you will be able to test and approve what God's will is—his good, pleasing and perfect will.
Romans 12:1–2

Like Dr. Rupe mentioned at the beginning of this chapter, no one can fully prepare for what pregnancy and having a baby entails. You can, however, do your best to get both your body and your mind in shape for the journey. You've spent some time with Dr. Rupe on the body, and now it's time to focus on your mind.

Our key Bible verse for this chapter talks about offering your body (or yourself) as a living sacrifice to God. If you are familiar with this verse, you know that this involves taking care of your body, as Dr. Rupe encourages. You may actually hate this verse. I know I did until I came to fully understand its meaning. I used to feel an overwhelming sense of failure when I read this verse. It says that in order to be a ready and worthy sacrifice, I must be holy and pleasing to God. But could I ever be truly holy and pleasing to God?

I came to understand that this instruction is not meant to bring pressure or condemnation on us but rather to encourage us to see ourselves and treat ourselves as a living sacrifice to God. Forget about what you see in the mirror daily that you wish you didn't see. You are a living sacrifice, cellulite and all. The next time you want to down a whole gallon of ice cream, remember that you are a living sacrifice. Viewing this sacrifice as your "spiritual act of worship" should empower you rather than discourage you. So whether you are beginning this journey in a very healthy place or starting out with a little more work to do, know that your very willingness to be diligent and do what is best for yourself and your future child is an act of worship.

I am definitely not the most diligent person in the world. Making the right food and exercise choices is usually overwhelming to me because I would choose to eat chocolate cake and not exercise whenever possible. If you are like me, it may be helpful to look at the process of choice—for your body, mind, or anything else for that matter—one choice at a time. As Dr. Rupe mentions in this chapter, it is important to plan ahead so that the right foods are available to you and so that exercise becomes a part of your routine. This planning will help you make better choices; however, you will still have to *choose* whether or not to exercise or to eat the right foods. When you encounter those moments of decision, remember that a healthy lifestyle is built one choice at a time. Try to make the best choice this time without thinking about the next time, and allow yourself some grace for those moments when ice cream may truly be the best choice for you. Remember that the key to a healthy lifestyle is balance.

Read the key verse again, this time in a different translation (Rom. 12:1–2 *The Message*).

> So here's what I want you to do, God helping you: Take your everyday, ordinary life—your sleeping, eating, going-to-work, and walking around life—and place it before God as an offering. Embracing what God does for you is the best thing you can do for him. Don't become so well-adjusted to your culture that you fit into it without even thinking. Instead, fix your attention on God. You'll be changed from the inside out. Readily recognize what he wants from you, and quickly respond to it. Unlike the culture around you, always dragging you down to its level of immaturity, God brings the best out of you, develops well-formed maturity in you.

I love this translation. Take every aspect of your life, especially the part where you desire to conceive a child, and place it before God. Then embrace what he does for you. It sounds so simple, yet it can still be challenging for some of us. But notice what the writer of *The Message* says before this instruction: "God helping you." We're not meant to do it in our own strength. He is there to help us every step of the way. This is true for every aspect of pregnancy and motherhood, so understanding and applying this truth now is going to help you along your entire journey.

The second half of our key verse talks about the mind. The *New International Version* says, "Do not conform . . . but be transformed by the renewing of your mind." What you are about to experience is absolutely mind-blowing. As you spend time trying to understand the miracle that is about to happen, you can turn to God's Word to refresh and renew your mind and to help you understand the reality of his greatness and his ability as demonstrated through the miracle of life. Simply focusing your attention to the One who is the Creator of life will bring all the peace and wisdom you need to travel this journey.

The last part of this passage says, "Then you will be able to test and approve what God's will is—his good, pleasing and perfect will." Here is clear instruction on how to know God's will. When you renew your mind on a daily basis, you will recognize his will. You will encounter some trials and many decisions along this road. If you are ready to handle them with a renewed mind, you might not lose yours.

Practical Ways to Renew Your Mind

It's easier said than done, right? You might be wondering how on earth you can renew your mind with so many thoughts and questions spinning around in your head. Ironically, those intrusions are exactly the reason you need to find strategies to renew your mind.

Read the Bible. This one might be obvious, but I wanted to reiterate the importance of filling your mind with truth in order to crowd out the stress and the fear. Try to find at least 15 minutes a day to sit quietly and meditate on what you are reading.

Read a book. Find an encouraging and inspirational book that will help you take a break from the pressures of life to refocus on a subject that you are passionate about or perhaps get lost in a really great fictional story.

Meditate. Grab a cup of decaf coffee or tea, sit somewhere you find peaceful and think about good things. Concentrate on the many blessings that surround you and thank God for them.

Recreate. Do something you enjoy. Shop, work out, explore nature. This method may not seem spiritual but I'd like to think that as long as I don't go crazy, God understands that I love shopping and hunting for bargains by myself. It completely renews my mind and spirit. If you hate to shop, go for a walk or knit a scarf. Whatever activity you enjoy, spend time on it when you need to refocus.

I want to take some time to address those of you who may be struggling to become pregnant. You will read more about my personal journey throughout this book, but I feel it is important to tell you here that my daughter did not come to us without a fight. I use the word *fight* because that is exactly what it was. After being diagnosed with polycystic ovary syndrome and, with it, infertility, two miscarriages, and countless pregnancy tests, I didn't think my dream of becoming a mother would ever come true. We prayed and believed and prayed some more. We rejoiced in our first two pregnancies and then grieved their losses. One Sunday at church, I actually moved to the other side of the congregation where all of the old people sat. I couldn't stand to be amid a sea of expectant moms (I think I once counted fifteen sitting around me). I trusted God and questioned God with the same longing heart, wondering if he would ever answer my cry for a child. A few years later he did—and it was well worth the wait.

I do not know your story, nor do I know how it will end, but I can tell you this: God knows your heart and he loves you. You may want to kick and scream every time you encounter a pregnant woman at the mall (I know I did). You may want to take a hiatus from church because you can't stand the sight of the mommies dropping their kids off at Sunday school. These are very valid emotions, and it's OK to feel them. But don't allow yourself to get caught up in the bitterness of waiting. Instead, allow God to renew your mind and prepare you for the unique journey he's planned for you. I've told many friends that sometimes I miss the sweetness that came with the sorrow of infertility. I miss the desperation that brought me closer to God. As hard as it might be to function as you wait for your longing to be fulfilled, be transformed by the renewing of your mind, and you will have all the peace and wisdom you need for your journey.

Do you feel ready to have a baby now? It's OK if the answer is still no. There's a lot more ground to cover, and we hope that with each new chapter of information and encouragement you'll feel a bit more at ease with the idea. Don't forget to refer back to the information in this chapter throughout your pregnancy. So much of what Dr. Rupe covers here applies to the months ahead. Take a moment now to pray through some common concerns at this stage, and write a prayer of your own for this time. We'll do this at the close of every chapter so that your entire journey will be covered in prayer. More than anything, we hope this process brings you closer to God.

Prayer Concerns

Wisdom to get your body ready

A renewed mind

Conception

Baby's early development

A Prayer for Your Journey

Dear Lord,

I want my body to be a living sacrifice, holy and pleasing to you. I know this will be the safest and most nurturing place for my child to be formed and to grow. Give me wisdom and strength to make the right choices daily. God, if there is anything in my body that would prevent or interfere with conception or pregnancy, I pray that you would heal me. I ask you to restore and renew my mind so that I will be able to discern your wisdom and know your will. Amen.

Write a prayer here for your own personal journey.

Journal

Record your thoughts and your fears here. It is important to acknowledge every thought and feeling you are experiencing. The main thing is to get them out in the open and, if they do not line up with the truth or the faith that you possess, get rid of those burdens by giving them over to your Pregnancy Companion.

Chapter Two

Am I Pregnant?
Weeks 1 to 5

Key Bible Verse

*Do not be anxious about anything, but in everything, by prayer
and petition, with thanksgiving, present your requests to God.
And the peace of God, which transcends all understanding, will guard your hearts and your minds in Christ Jesus.*

Philippians 4:6–7

Finding out you are pregnant can be one of the most exciting events in your life. It can also be one of the scariest. It's completely normal if you feel both emotions. Get used to that mixture now, as you'll likely feel it regularly as you experience pregnancy, childbirth, baby's first steps, the first day of school, junior high, graduation . . . you get the idea. As we dig into all the new information you will need for this journey, remember to invite peace to take over your heart and mind so that it can push fear out.

Baby Stats

So how far along are you? This is one of the most confusing things about early pregnancy. Traditionally, people refer to pregnancy in months, saying it takes nine to make a baby. Medically, however, we actually describe pregnancy in weeks. Doctors use a forty-week timeline, which is . . . yes, you guessed it, closer to ten months. It's confusing, I know. Patients always ask me how many months pregnant they are, and I try to translate their weeks to months as best I can. So, for the sake of accuracy, in this book we will follow pregnancy in weeks, not months.

Your due date and your gestational weeks are determined by the ever-important first day of your last menstrual period (FDLMP). Hopefully you were tracking this as we discussed it in Chapter One. The counting of gestational weeks begins at the FDLMP. At this point, anyone with even a basic understanding of biology is probably getting a furrowed brow. If you don't even ovulate until the midpoint of your cycle, why do you start counting "pregnancy weeks" with your last period? I wish I had a good answer for you. It doesn't make sense, and it's a bit confusing, but that's the way it's done. Accepting this oddity will help you make sense of the math throughout your pregnancy. How's that for clear-cut information?

Ovulation and Implantation

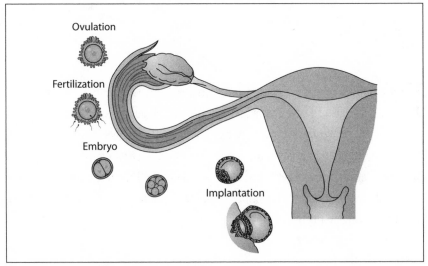

© 2010 Wolters Kluwer Health | Lippincott Williams and Wilkins

Ovulation occurs approximately fourteen days after the FDLMP. The ovaries spit out an egg (or sometimes two) into the abdomen. The fallopian tubes pick up the egg so it can journey to the inside of the uterus. It is in the fallopian tube that the egg is fertilized, that is, if there are any good lookin' sperm around. The majority of eggs *do* get fertilized. The tricky part is getting those fertilized eggs to attach to the uterus. Only about thirty percent of them will attach and begin to grow. During this time, the baby is made up of only one hundred cells. It grows rapidly, going from hundreds of cells to millions of cells in only a matter of weeks. This rapid cell growth is the reason you need the good nutrition we discussed in Chapter One, especially the folic acid, which is essential for the backbone of baby's DNA.

As the baby begins to grow, it secretes a hormone called human chorionic growth hormone (HCG). This hormone is what makes a pregnancy test read positive. A test that you buy at the drug store will usually be positive at an HCG level of about 50. So when you miss your period, you take a test and if it's positive, you're pregnant. You typically do not need a blood test or a urine test at the doctor's office to confirm a positive home test, unless you are high-risk and your doctor has instructed you to take one. Over-the-counter tests are quite accurate; however, if you get a negative result, it is possible that your levels aren't quite high enough to show in your urine yet. If the test is negative and you still don't start your period a few days later, then take another.

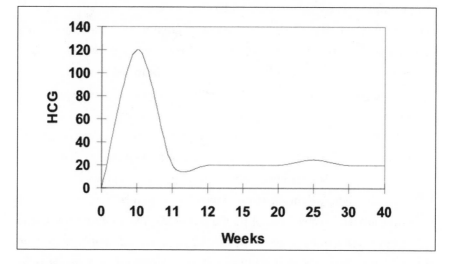

When you miss your first period and have a positive pregnancy test, you are about four weeks pregnant. The baby itself has only been implanted for two weeks, so essentially the forty-week measurement system for pregnancy gives you a two-week jumpstart.

Mommy Stats

Even though there are a zillion things going on at a cellular level, there are not too many changes that will be physically apparent in you just yet. As your progesterone levels increase and your HCG levels increase, you may feel your breasts enlarging and becoming more sensitive. Some people will experience nausea, although this symptom comes more commonly at eight weeks.

When You're Sick

Being sick when you're already miserable from pregnancy can be a double yuck! Your immune system is not as strong during pregnancy, so chances are you will have some amount of illness during your pregnancy. The key is to rest, stay hydrated, and let your doctor know if you're not improving quickly.

Stomach flu can be especially nasty during pregnancy. Ironically, it seems to hit right after people get over morning sickness. I often hear, "I thought I was done with all this!" Try to keep fluids such as Gatorade down. It is safe to take loperamide (Imodium) for diarrhea, or if you were given nausea medicine for your morning sickness, you can take that as well. If you ever have vomiting or diarrhea for more than twenty-four hours straight, you need to seek medical attention because you could get dehydrated. This is not good for you or baby.

Colds and upper respiratory illnesses are also quite annoying. Acetaminophen (Tylenol), guaifenesin (Robitussin), and phenylephrine (Sudafed) are generally safe to take during pregnancy. Make sure to avoid products that contain ibuprofen (Motrin or Advil) or aspirin. If you begin to cough up chunky junk (yes, that's a medical term) or have a fever, you should see your doctor. It is highly recommended that you get the flu shot while you are pregnant. If you do get influenza with body aches, chills, and fevers, you should be started on antiviral drugs quickly. Some OB offices treat their sick pregnant patients in the office; others will have you see your family doctor. Check with your doctor on office policy.

Urinary tract infections (UTIs) are very common during pregnancy, which is one of the reasons that you have to give a urine sample *every* time you visit your OB. If you experience burning, pain, or frequent urination (more than normal), start yourself on cranberry juice and call your doctor right away. If you are being treated with antibiotics for an infection and the symptoms are not getting better, let your doctor know. Also notify her if you begin to have fever or back pain; these could be signs the infection is spreading from your bladder to your kidney, which can be very serious during pregnancy.

Illness	Do	Don't
Common cold Upper respiratory infection	• Rest • Drink fluids • Take acetaminophen (Tylenol), guaifenesin (Robitussin), phenylephrine (Sudafed) • Call your doctor with fever, trouble breathing, or coughing up mucus • Use Vicks VapoRub	• Take meds with ibuprofen or aspirin • Drink a hot toddy or medicines containing alcohol
Influenza	• Get the flu shot to prevent it • Drink fluids • Rest • Take loperamide (Imodium) for diarrhea • Take antiviral drugs prescribed by doctor	• Take meds with ibuprofen or aspirin • Get dehydrated • Drink a hot toddy or medicines containing alcohol
Urinary tract infection	• See your doctor immediately • Drink cranberry juice • Take antibiotics prescribed by doctor	• Just "wait" and drink cranberry juice • Take meds with ibuprofen or aspirin

Symptom Checker

In each chapter, we will list common symptoms you may be experiencing at this stage in pregnancy. Please remember that you may experience some, all, or none of these symptoms.

☐ Fatigue   ☐ Nausea   ☐ Did I mention fatigue?
☐ Swollen breasts ☐ Increased urination

A good thing to remember about pregnancy in general and *especially* the first few months of pregnancy is that everybody is different. Some people are very in tune with their bodies and can tell you which ovary they ovulated from that month. Other people have no clue what's going on with their cycles. Some women "feel" pregnant right away; others don't have the classic first trimester symptoms until closer to ten weeks. A lot of women still feel pretty normal throughout the entire pregnancy and really cherish the time. I encourage these women not to talk too loudly in our waiting room, or the sick ones might beat them up in the parking lot. Try not to compare yourself to your girlfriend or the lady in the next cubicle at work. Especially don't let your mom stress you out because you're not puking the first day you pee on a stick and see double pink lines.

You may have some cramping and mild pelvic pain. *Wait! Did you say pain? I thought pain was bad!* Yes and no. Remember when I explained that the ovary spits out the egg? What that actually means is that the egg dissolves a hole in the ovary to escape. The fluid surrounding the egg begins to swell and forms a cyst that produces the hormone (progesterone) that helps the baby grow. That swollen ovary can cause some cramping pain. The uterus is made entirely of muscle, and as this muscle grows with the baby, there can also be some cramping sensations. If cramping is severe, then you should call your doctor. There are a lot of strange aches and pains associated with pregnancy. With each painful sensation, it's hard to keep your mind from going to the worst-case scenario. I often see patients near tears with complaints of pain. By the time I get the chance to ask how bad the pain is, they tell me it's gone. The nervous mother-to-be is usually sure that pain so intense just had to hurt the baby, even though it only lasted a minute. Here's a good rule to go by. If something serious is happening, then the pain is going to last longer than a couple of minutes or happen more than once. So relax. Don't get all worked up by every little ache and pain. If you do, you'll spend the majority of your pregnancy stressed out.

And then there is spotting. Rightfully so, most women seem to freak out about spotting. When the embryo implants into the lining of the uterus, it literally invades these cells. The cells that line the uterus have tons of blood flow going to them, so the baby is like a leech that taps into this maternal blood supply for its nutrition and growth. The more it grows, the more it invades. Then it forms the placenta. The placenta is a disk-shaped organ that attaches to the uterus and transfers nutrition to the baby via the umbilical cord. With as much blood that flows to the lining of the uterus and then into the baby, it's amazing that there isn't more bleeding in pregnancy. Statistically, about ten percent of women will have some amount of spotting in the first trimester. However, bleeding can also be a sign that something is wrong. So, what's an emotional pregnant girl to do when she sees the dreaded color red on her toilet paper?

The most common time for spotting is about when you would have had a period. This is when implantation is in full force. If the spotting is a small amount of brown discharge that happens only once or twice while using the restroom, it's usually just implantation, and you'll need to wait and see. If the bleeding becomes red or requires a pad or is accompanied by pain, then you should call your doctor.

But Dr. Rupe, I'm a nervous wreck. I don't want to "wait and see." I called my doctor, and she said there was nothing she could do. The time between your missed period and your first doctor's visit can seem like an eternity for some people, especially if you have a history of miscarriage. As doctors, we are trained to fix things. That means that if there really is something wrong at four to six weeks, we honestly can't do anything to save the pregnancy. What we can do is offer information and reassurance. Before five weeks, it's too early to see anything on ultrasound; however, we can check HCG levels to make sure they are normal. (See HCG graph.) Remember hormone levels go up daily, so we can look at the levels over time to make sure they are rising appropriately. If you are really worried, you can ask to have your levels checked to put your mind at ease. But even before you do that—stop, take a deep breath, and pray that God will protect you and your baby.

Risk Factors for Tubal (Ectopic) Pregnancy

Previous ectopic pregnancy
History of surgery on your tubes
Getting pregnant after having tubes tied
History of pelvic inflammatory disease
Endometriosis

Ectopic Pregnancy

Another reason to notify your doctor of increasing pain is the possibility of ectopic pregnancy (tubal pregnancy). In an ectopic pregnancy, the embryo implants not in the lining of the uterus where it is supposed to be, but instead somewhere else in the pelvis, most commonly in the fallopian tube. As the embryo begins to grow, it will do two distinct things. It causes the tube to swell, and it begins to invade the blood vessels of the tube. This usually causes pain. If the ectopic pregnancy is discovered early, your doctor may opt to give you a shot that can help dissolve it. Oftentimes we don't discover ectopics until they grow so big that they break open the tube (called rupturing). This causes severe pain and dizziness, can lead to life-threatening internal bleeding, and was a leading cause of death associated with pregnancy until the late nineteenth century.

Less than two percent of pregnancies are found to be ectopic, and even with modern technology, five percent of those cases can be life-threatening. When pain in early pregnancy gets worse and not better with acetaminophen or rest, then notify your doctor. It is also important to realize that by removing an ectopic pregnancy, you are in no way committing abortion. This pregnancy has no chance of survival. There is no technology that can move the embryo into the uterus. It can only cause harm to you and your reproductive organs. This possibility may seem scary and overwhelming, but also be assured that with prompt medical attention, it can usually be resolved quickly.

Expectations for This Month's Visit

Most OB offices do not schedule your first visit until seven to eight weeks into your pregnancy. Definitely call right away to get your appointment, though, and be prepared for the staff to ask for your FDLMP when scheduling. If you are not already on prenatal vitamins, you can ask the office to call in a prescription to get you started before your appointment.

During this time, it may be helpful to prepare a list of questions for your doctor. There may even be some questions and symptoms that you want to ask about before your first regularly scheduled visit. If you are taking medication, then you should check with the office to make sure it's safe to continue them in pregnancy. If you are at a high risk for tubal pregnancy, inform the office when you make your appointment because they will want to see you sooner. If you have persistent or severe pain or signs of dehydration before your scheduled visit, call your doctor or go to the emergency room.

Signs of Dehydration

Weight loss
Dark-colored urine
Dry mouth
Vomiting more than twelve hours straight
Feeling dizzy or light-headed

Choosing a Doctor

Picking a doctor or midwife is a big decision with many factors to consider. Some patients will already be established with an OB, so they can just discuss how pregnancies are handled at their annual exam. If you are not established, it's nice to meet with the doctor before pregnancy to see if she makes you feel comfortable and to get a feel for how the practice operates. For patients who are high risk, you will want to discuss any issues with your physician before pregnancy.

You want to find a doctor who accepts your insurance and delivers at a hospital that also accepts your insurance. If you are high risk, you should make sure that the hospital has a neonatal intensive care unit (NICU). Next, consider how the practice handles patients when their doctor is not available. Some practices only share on-call duties within their group, while some will share the load with other groups. If this is the case, you may find yourself in labor with a doctor you've never met before. If the practice shares responsibility within their group, ask whether you will have the opportunity to meet the other doctors who might deliver your baby. Some women are adamant about who they want to deliver their baby. Others couldn't care less as long as they get that baby out! Simply make sure you are comfortable with every possible scenario.

High Risk?

High-risk pregnancies are those with a higher chance of things going wrong, such as preterm delivery or stillbirth. High-risk pregnancies include twins, placenta previa, and preterm labor. Having a medical condition such as diabetes, hypertension, or epilepsy may also make you high risk. More information on high-risk factors can be found in Chapter Ten.

A certified nurse-midwife (CNM) is a nurse who has received additional training in childbirth and postpartum care. CNMs are licensed and practice in all fifty states in the United States. They practice on a nursing model with special focus on natural childbirth. Midwives cannot do cesarean sections or handle high-risk pregnancies, so they usually practice in collaboration with physicians. Midwives are a great option for low-risk pregnancies. They are often able to devote more time to patient education and are able to spend more time with patients during labor.

Some patients place a lot of emphasis on the gender of their provider. I get many patients who say they prefer a female OB because "they understand" better what women go through. While I appreciate the business and try to be the best, most compassionate physician I can be, I honestly feel that—as with any other physical attribute—you shouldn't choose your doctor based on gender alone. Some of the best OBs I work with have been male. They can at times be more compassionate than female OBs. When I have a patient who is constantly complaining about the discomfort of pregnancy, I try to be compassionate and supportive. But I admit that in the back of my mind I'm sometimes thinking, "Yes, I know pregnancy is uncomfortable because I worked twelve-hour days right up to and including the day I delivered my son!"

Most importantly, you want a doctor who will really listen to you, is board certified in his or her field, and with whom you feel comfortable. You can ask for recommendations from friends or co-workers. The best way to find a quality OB is to call the labor and delivery unit at your local hospital and ask the charge nurse which doctor she would recommend. No one knows the OB doctors better than the labor and delivery nurses.

Provider Checklist

- ☐ Are they board certified?
- ☐ Do they accept my insurance?
- ☐ Do they deliver at a hospital that takes my insurance?
- ☐ Are the office hours convenient? (This is especially important for working women.)
- ☐ Is the location convenient?
- ☐ Will I talk to the doctor or a nurse if I call with non-emergency questions?
- ☐ Is the office organized? Are calls returned promptly?

So what happens if halfway through the pregnancy, you begin to feel your doctor is not the right fit? If you feel uncomfortable with your doctor, then strongly consider changing practices. If you do feel the need to change providers, you should do so before thirty-five weeks, because most practices won't accept new patients after this time.

Tips for Communicating with Doctors and Nurses

Make lists. Be it your pregnancy brain or the hectic nature of your day, you are likely to forget a few of your questions if you don't write them down before your visit. Use your smartphone or keep a notepad with you through the week to jot down questions as you think of them. Start with your most important questions first. Your doctor may not have time to answer every question at every visit, especially for patients who bring in pages (plural) of questions. Most days I can spend as much time as I need to with my patients to get their questions answered. Occasionally, I may have had a delivery or an emergency surgery that has put me behind. I may ask the patient if any non-emergency questions can be answered at the next visit or if I can call her at the end of the day.

Be direct. If you have specific concerns, don't beat around the bush. Just say what's on your mind. I don't mean to be rude, of course, but I find that patients will often be embarrassed about their questions or concerns and become evasive. Or they worry about my reaction to their question. Trust me, we've heard everything, and there is no such thing as a dumb question. That is to say, if it concerns you enough to write it down, it's not a dumb question to you.

Take your physician's advice! If you don't agree with your physician's advice, then let her know. Probably the most frustrating thing to me as a doctor is when patients do not follow my recommendations—and then they don't tell me. It's OK to disagree with your doctor, just let her know so you can come up with a plan that both of you agree on. For example, I've had a pregnant patient whose urine showed signs of infection, she didn't take her antibiotics, and she didn't tell me. Then she ended up with a more severe kidney infection. When I asked her why, she said that she wasn't having any symptoms, so she thought it was early enough to just treat with cranberry juice. Plus, she was worried about getting a yeast infection. If I had known, I could have given her an antibiotic that didn't cause a yeast infection and explained the importance of taking the medication. If she had still chosen not to take it, I could have monitored her more closely for worsening symptoms.

I've also had patients who told me they quit smoking when they really didn't. I ran into one of my patients smoking outside the grocery store once! Be sure your sins will find you out, especially in a small town. So if you can't kick the habit, your doctor needs to know so that she can pay special attention to signs that the smoking is causing complications.

Be prepared when calling the doctor's office. When you call with a routine question, you will most likely be asked to leave a message. You may also be asked to leave your pharmacy's number, so it's a good idea to have it handy before calling. Also, after you leave a message, keep your phone with you so the office can call you back. If you leave a cell phone number, make sure your battery is charged. It's best to call first thing in the morning. If you are calling with an emergent question, let the office know that you need to speak with someone quickly.

Planning Ahead

This is a good time to look at your life plans for the next year. Having a baby is a major life change, so you should try, if possible, to limit other life changes this year. Moving, job changes, a wedding or divorce should be avoided. If you don't really have control over these changes, aim to complete any major life change before week thirty of your pregnancy. If you are planning a vacation, taking it in the second trimester (between weeks thirteen and twenty-four) is usually best. That's when you feel the best and the risk of complications is low. Additionally, if your job involves travel, you will not want to plan any trips after thirty-five weeks.

Common Questions You May Have This Month

I was on the pill when I got pregnant. Is that going to hurt my baby?
No. There is no evidence that being on the pill can cause birth defects. Obviously discontinue the pill when you find out you are pregnant, and let your provider know at your initial visit about all medications that you have taken during pregnancy.

I don't feel like I did in my last pregnancy. Is everything OK?
Most likely yes. Each pregnancy is different. It is common for people to be nauseated with one pregnancy and feel great the next. It also seems that with second pregnancies, patients have more discomfort and cramping in the beginning. Don't worry if this pregnancy is different than your last. A different life is growing inside you. This is just the beginning of how different things are going to be! Talk to your doctor about any specific concerns you have.

I don't have regular menstrual cycles. How do I know how far along I am?
If your cycles are irregular, then the best way to know is by getting an early ultrasound. You can first see a heartbeat at six weeks of pregnancy. Let your doctor know your cycle length and when your pregnancy test was first positive.

Do my eating habits affect the baby's eating preferences later in life?
There is no evidence that says if you crave apples during pregnancy, your child will later like apples. However, as the child develops, he will learn his eating habits by watching his parents, so continuing with healthy habits as the baby gets older is extremely important.

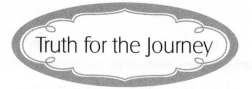
Truth for the Journey

Do not be anxious about anything, but in everything, by prayer and petition, with thanksgiving, present your requests to God. And the peace of God, which transcends all understanding, will guard your hearts and your minds in Christ Jesus.
Philippians 4:6–7

By now, your head probably hurts from the math you've had to do this month. It can be confusing trying to figure out your due date. Ask your doctor if she has one of those little wheels in the office that figures your due date for you, and then go with it. Trust me, it's an estimate so just go with what the wheel says. Perhaps you are reading this after discovering you did not conceive this month. Don't get me started on how that can make your head *and* your heart hurt. I want to address the myriad emotions you may be experiencing at this point.

Our key verse for this month says not to be anxious about anything but to pray about the concerns of your heart. Do you feel anxious? If you just discovered you are pregnant, are you worried about your baby? If you did not conceive this month, are you concerned that it will never happen? As if a woman's hormones weren't enough to deal with, add in the hoping and waiting, and forget it—we're a mess! But we don't have to be. You may already be intimately familiar with this verse, but just because we know something doesn't mean we apply it to our lives. So let's just assume there is some level of anxiety going on in you at this point. What are you going to do about it? Paul instructs in this verse that when we are anxious, we should pray and petition the Lord. Lay your thoughts and fears before him, but don't forget to do it with thanksgiving.

I've often wondered why the word *thanksgiving* is used here. It's almost like he dropped it in there after the fact. I believe it's there to offer us balance. The God of Heaven is always available to hear the dreams and desires of our hearts. But how selfish it would be of us to ask, ask, and ask some more without ever giving him thanksgiving and praise. We need to be ready to *thank* him first and *ask* him second. *The Message* actually says, "Let petitions and praises shape your worries into prayers." Wow. What an amazing way to look at worry. As you think about all the things that are making you sweat right now (besides the hormones, that is), take a moment to thank God for all of the good things he has done in your life. Then begin to share the details that are invading your mind. Your honesty and your thankful heart can shape those worries into prayers. His Word promises that he will give you an incredible peace that transcends all understanding.

As Dr. Rupe said, this is a crucial time for baby's early development. What happens with your baby during the first few weeks might seem minor since you cannot see or feel it. Actually, there is a major miracle going on inside of you. Instead of focusing on what can go wrong, purpose to turn your thoughts to the amazing miracle of life. Every time you think of something scary that could happen, replace that thought with the truth of all that is going right. Perhaps you aren't dealing with worry at all at this point. If that is the case, then I encourage you to share your peace with others around you. Your life can be an example of the fruit of knowing God.

When you are infertile with irregular periods, there's no telling how long you should wait to take a pregnancy test. When I was trying to conceive, I kept taking them, each time a roller coaster of emotion, hoping and waiting and being disappointed yet again. I am likely one of many girls who should have bought stock in First Response. I cannot count how many sticks I've peed on thus far in my childbearing years. I know now that I should have more often accessed the peace that was always available to me.

Each of us has our own story that God is writing for our family. We all come from different backgrounds and have different circumstances surrounding our pregnancies. I hope that no matter what your story is, you are able to tap into the sweet peace of God throughout your journey. Whether you are excited to be pregnant, have been trying for a long time with no results, or are dreading the positive result that seems imminent, you can have peace as your unique story is written.

Prayer Concerns
Baby's early development
A thankful heart
Pure peace

A Prayer for Your Journey

Dear Lord,

Thank you for the incredible blessings you have given me. A baby will be another example of your great goodness. Help me God to focus on you as I continue this process. I trust you to develop my baby perfectly from head to toes. Grant me the wisdom and peace you promised in your Word as I present my requests to you. I thank you in advance for these things. Amen.

Write a prayer here for your own personal journey.

_____

_____

_____

_____

_____

Journal

Record your thoughts and your fears here. It is important to acknowledge every thought and feeling you are experiencing. The main thing is to get them out in the open, and if they do not line up with the truth or the faith that you possess, then get rid of those burdens by giving them over to your Pregnancy Companion.

_____

_____

_____

_____

_____

Chapter Three

Great Expectations
Weeks 6 to 10

Key Bible Verse

Many, O Lord My God, are the wonders you have done. The things you planned for us no one can recount to you; were I to speak and tell of them, they would be too many to declare.

Psalms 40:5

Baby Stats

Your baby is about ⅓ of an inch long at six weeks. That's approximately the size of your fingertip. Baby's little heart is already beating between 120 and 170 beats per minute. This is a stage of rapid growth, with the baby being 1¼ inches long (crown to rump) by ten weeks' gestation. This month, baby is growing from the size of a small peanut to a grape.

At this point, all of baby's organs are forming, and all his little pieces and parts are coming together. A few things are known to cause malformations at this stage of development. One of them is extreme heat. This is a time when it is especially essential to avoid hot tubs or very hot baths (higher than body temperature). Having a high core temperature at this stage of pregnancy has been shown to cause malformation of the spinal cord. If you have a fever at this time, it is best to take acetaminophen (Tylenol) to help keep your temperature down. If that does not lower your temperature, then call

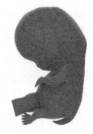

your doctor. Do not stress about being out in the hot sun for a few hours or taking a hot shower. I'm referring to extended amounts of very high temperature.

The other main source of malformations is medication. Be cautious of taking any medications that might interfere with the development of the baby. Check with your doctor before taking any medication: prescription, over-the-counter, herbal supplements, and/or additional vitamins. Ibuprofen (Advil or Motrin) is not recommended in pregnancy, although it is most harmful if taken in the third trimester.

Dangerous Medications

Medications/substances that are known to cause fetal malformations include:

Accutane	Valproic acid
Coumadin	Cocaine
ACE inhibitors	Tamoxifen
Lithium	Thalidomide

You should also be cautious of chemicals during pregnancy. If your job requires you to handle harsh chemicals (in a lab setting, for example), then you need to speak with your doctor about the specific precautions you should take. You may be wondering if coloring your hair or getting a spray tan will affect your baby's development. Or what about household cleaning supplies? Hair dye has not been proven to cause malformations because it is minimally absorbed by the skin. Coloring your hair is considered safe, but if you want to be overly cautious, you can wait until you are twelve weeks along. But beware: my friend the hairdresser says that hair color sometimes "takes differently" in expectant moms due to the hormonal changes of pregnancy.

Self-tanning lotions are also minimally absorbed and are considered safe to use. We recommend you stay away from tanning beds in general, and this applies during pregnancy as well. The light from the tanning bed doesn't penetrate through the skin, but there is concern that the high temperatures in the tanning beds could have the same effect as hot tubs and interfere with the neural tube development of the baby.

Regular cleaning supplies are fine (sorry, I can't give you an excuse to get out of your housekeeping). Just make sure you keep all areas well ventilated while cleaning. Avoid solvents such as paint thinner. Use common sense: if a chemical requires specialized disposal, you probably shouldn't handle it while you are pregnant.

Most cosmetics and lotions are safe—with the exception of Retin-A, which you should discontinue during pregnancy. If you have questions about any prescription lotions, ask your doctor. On the other hand, I once had a patient bring in three grocery bags full of every toiletry in her house for me to inspect and make sure they were safe for pregnancy. Yes, deodorant, toothpaste, and shampoo are all safe for your baby. There is no need to bring your doctor every household and personal item for inspection. If you have a question about something you use, simply ask about it at your next visit.

Mommy Stats

At this point, you may not be able to look in the mirror and see any obvious signs of pregnancy . . . that is, until you look at your face, where you will probably be looking a little squeamish. We'll discuss nausea in more detail in the next section, Symptom Checker.

I want to address everyone's favorite pregnancy subject: weight gain. It always seems like women approach weight gain during pregnancy in one of two ways. I'm going to eat everything in sight (Woo hoo! I'm pregnant! I can eat whatever I want!) OR I'm terrified of getting fat (let me inspect the scale daily and check constantly for stretch marks).

The balance of course is somewhere in the middle.

Pregnancy weight gain should be based on prepregnancy weight. Refer to BMI chart in Appendix to determine your BMI if you have not already done so. Those with a normal weight (BMI of 20–26) should aim for a weight gain of twenty-five to thirty-five pounds. Underweight women (BMI < 20) should try to gain thirty to forty pounds. Overweight women (BMI 26–29) should aim for fifteen to twenty-five pounds. Obese individuals (BMI > 30) should gain less than fifteen pounds and may actually lose weight during pregnancy once they start on a healthier diet. If you are vertically challenged (under 63 inches), it is recommended to try to stay on the lower end of normal weight gain.

Before twenty weeks the baby weighs very little; until that time, your weight gain goal should be one to five pounds. Then try to keep weight gain to approximately a pound a week thereafter. There are usually months when you don't gain any weight followed by those during which you may gain ten pounds. I try to encourage people to look at the overall picture and not get too wrapped up in the scale changes with each visit. If you are continuing to gain too little or too much weight, you may need to meet with a nutritionist. Don't get overwhelmed and just throw in the towel because it seems too complicated.

Weight Gain Recommendations {According to your BMI}	
BMI	Appropriate Weight Gain
Less than 20	30-40 lbs
20-26	25-35 lbs
26-29	15-25 lbs
30 or more	Up to 15 lbs

During pregnancy, you only need about three hundred extra calories per day. *So you are not eating for two!* You are eating for one and one sixth! Review the section in Chapter One on nutrition in pregnancy and the sample menus included. Try to eat an overall balanced diet. If you follow these five rules the majority of the time, then you're going to be doing great.

- Five servings of fruits and vegetables (try to make at least one of them green)
- Eight glasses (64 ounces) of water
- Whole grains
- Protein with each meal
- Prenatal vitamin

Financial Resources

The government program for women, infants, and children (WIC) is a great resource for mothers who earn a low income. It provides free, nutritious food during pregnancy and postpartum, as well as education and breastfeeding support. Some local WIC offices even provide breast pumps. If you are financially challenged, please check out the WIC office nearest you to see if you qualify. You can find a list of phone numbers at www.fns.usda.gov/wic.

During pregnancy, your immune system is not as strong as it usually is, making you more prone to illness. Take caution to avoid being around sick people, if possible. Wash hands thoroughly with soap and water for thirty seconds before meals and after using the restroom. Carry lots of hand sanitizer. The influenza vaccine is recommended in pregnancy.

Symptom Checker

☐ Morning sickness (nausea)   ☐ Hunger (with cravings and aversions)
☐ Fatigue   ☐ Dizziness
☐ Frequent urination   ☐ Breast tenderness
☐ Constipation

Nausea. The majority of women will experience at least occasional nausea during the first trimester, with about two percent experiencing severe daily vomiting that we refer to as *hyperemesis gravidarum*. As a starting strategy, eat small meals throughout the day and stop before you are full. Keep crackers beside your bed so you can eat them before you get up in the morning. Getting up very slowly can also be helpful.

Some women will encounter specific foods or smells that trigger nausea. If you know what foods are troublesome for you, plan ahead to avoid them. In general, steer clear of spicy, rich, or fried foods. Other women will experience nausea brushing their teeth (but please don't avoid this one!) or with activities like pumping gas.

If the nausea is not improving, the next step would be to take a combination of vitamin B6 (10 mg) and the antihistamine doxylamine (Unisom, 10 mg) every six hours as needed. These are safe and available over the counter. Obviously, the antihistamine may make you tired, but it does help the nausea. Natural ginger supplements have been shown in some studies to reduce nausea. If you're still vomiting regularly or find your nausea incapacitating, then please call your doctor's office. There are several safe prescription medications that can help you manage the nausea.

Whatever you do, don't stop taking your prenatal vitamins! I see lots of patients whose vitamins make them throw up, so they stop taking them. If your vitamin causes nausea, notify your doctor so she can prescribe a different brand. If you still can't tolerate them, then at least keep taking the folic acid, which is essential at this point in pregnancy.

A few of you probably laughed out loud at the short list of daily recommended foods I mentioned earlier in this chapter. You might think at this point in pregnancy that just holding down a milkshake is an accomplishment. For those of you struggling with nausea, try to do the best you can. Foods like whole grain toast or bagels, applesauce, bananas, yogurt, and brown rice are better choices than white bread and ice cream. Most people can still navigate their nausea and aversions to maintain a generally balanced diet. I did have a patient who could eat only bagels without throwing up. I remember her nearly in tears as she described her Thanksgiving dinner consisting only of a bagel. In these extreme situations, additional nutritional evaluations may need to be made. This can be the most difficult time to keep your nutritional balance, but still try to focus on getting as many fruits and vegetables as possible.

But what about the cravings? Some cravings are good. If you are craving a specific fruit, then go with it. If you need a Hershey's bar every afternoon, then you may need to slow down. I tell patients to give in to their "bad" cravings once or twice a week—not once or twice a day!

There are weird cravings that could be the signal that something abnormal is going on. For instance, if you crave plain ice all the time, you could be anemic. Also, some women will crave dirt or laundry soap, as well as other non-foods. Such cravings could be signaling specific vitamin deficiencies. If this is the case, inform your doctor.

Fatigue. And then there's the fatigue. I think fatigue is the least-discussed early pregnancy symptom. Everybody knows about the morning sickness, but sometimes fatigue can be the most debilitating symptom in early pregnancy. The source is thought to be a combination of the high levels of HCG and progesterone but—whatever causes it—most pregnant women just want to sleep from about six weeks to twelve weeks. Like twelve hours a night . . . and then take a nap during the day. Fatigue and nausea seem to get better after twelve weeks, but the combination of the two can be quite concerning. On several occasions, I've had husbands pull me aside and say things like, "I'm really worried about my wife. All she wants to do is sleep. No, really, all the time! Is she OK?" I tell them that it is normal and encourage them to let her rest as much as she can. The tiredness usually improves as the second trimester begins. However, I leave them with the warning that fatigue may return in the last six weeks of pregnancy as well.

Expectations for This Month's Visit

This is usually the first visit to your OB after you've become pregnant. At this appointment, you may have an ultrasound (sonogram). If you do, you'll see that the baby looks like a tiny, blinking dot at six weeks of gestation. By ten weeks, though, the baby will look like a little, wiggly person with arms and legs. An ultrasound at this point in pregnancy is done vaginally—the best way to see the baby at this stage. Now, the vaginal probe on the ultrasound machine can look a little (OK, a lot) intimidating the first time you see it. But its diameter is smaller than the speculum used for a Pap smear and is also smaller than the thing that got you pregnant in the first place. So relax. The vaginal ultrasound should not be painful. If it is, tell the provider. Once you have seen a heartbeat on ultrasound, the risk of miscarriage is less than ten percent, so this is very reassuring.

Your doctor will probably do a Pap smear and cultures to test for infection. Blood will be drawn to determine your blood type, check for anemia, and look for other signs of diseases such as hepatitis and HIV. These tests are all standard and some are required by state law. So your doctor is not ordering a gonorrhea test because she thinks you have it, it's just part of the protocol.

One other thing that you will do at this visit—well, actually at *every* visit—is pee. There is a whole lotta peeing in a cup going on at the OB office. This is primarily because in pregnancy you are more prone to urinary tract infections for several reasons. One reason is the weak immune system we mentioned earlier. Another is that increased progesterone levels can relax the valves in your bladder, which increases your risk of getting a UTI. Bladder infections can lead to kidney infections, which are also more serious in pregnancy because they may lead to preterm labor and other serious complications. At times you can have an infection without symptoms, which is why we check every visit. You may also have protein in your urine, a sign that your kidneys aren't functioning properly and a symptom of preeclampsia, which we will discuss in Chapter Ten. Preeclampsia is a complication that can happen toward the end of pregnancy (so don't worry about it now!).

Your doctor will ask questions about your family history at your first visit. Some offices will utilize a nurse practitioner for this visit. These questions are intended to check for possible risks for the genetic disorders we discussed in Chapter One. I always feel like the Red Cross lady during this part of the exam, as if I were asking all those crazy questions so my patient can give blood. Your doctor should also go over a list of pregnancy restrictions.

Lifting. During pregnancy, you are more prone to injury. You are off balance due to your belly, and your joints are looser. Mainly for these reasons, we restrict lifting to less than forty pounds. Lifting does not hurt the baby or cause miscarriage. We are simply trying to help you avoid injury during pregnancy.

Alcohol. There is no known safe amount of alcohol in pregnancy. That being said, sixty percent of all pregnancies are unplanned, so I often get questions from women who drank early in their pregnancy. They may not have realized they were pregnant and were concerned that their baby could have fetal alcohol syndrome. Fetal alcohol syndrome is associated with physical deformities as well as mental retardation. It is most commonly associated with women who drink regularly as well as binge drink during their entire pregnancy. It is rarely, if ever, reported from occasional drinking in the first trimester. This is not meant to give you permission to drink but to help alleviate the fears of those who drank alcohol before realizing they were pregnant.[1]

Fish. As we mentioned in Chapter One, larger ocean fish can have elevated levels of mercury that may be harmful in pregnancy. Fish does contain DHA, which is essential for brain development, so two servings of smaller, low-mercury fish (like salmon or trout) can be eaten per week.

Foods associated with listeria. I recently got a frantic, after-hours call that went something like this: "Oh no! I just ate deli meat. Then later I was reading my pregnancy book, and it said it was really dangerous! Is my baby going to die?" The short answer is, "No." Listeria is bacteria that can cause infection in immuno-compromised individuals such as the young, the elderly, and you guessed it . . . the pregnant. There have been outbreaks of listeria associated with various foods including raw vegetables, processed foods such as hot dogs, deli meats, unpas-teurized cider, and milk. The infection can be very severe in the mom and baby and lead to bad stuff like preterm delivery or even stillbirth. Yes, it sounds scary, but the actual incidence of listeria is the U.S. is extremely rare. According to the Centers for Disease Control and Prevention (CDC), the rate of listeria infection in the U.S. is one person per nine hundred thousand.[2]

Your chance of having a life-threatening case of the flu during pregnancy is only one in a thousand. Now that's not meant to scare you about the flu, it's just meant to put things in perspective. I've seen patients avoid lunch meat and all possible foods that might be associated with listeria and then refuse their flu shot for "safety concerns." The best intervention for both is common sense. Wash your hands thoroughly with soap and water before you eat. Make sure all raw vegeta-bles are washed and clean. Items such as bean sprouts that are difficult to wash should be avoided.

Be cautious of deli meat. If you are at a party and the tray of deli meat has been sitting out, don't eat it. Same goes for hot dogs. Avoid unpasteurized cheese, juice, and milk (remember that some organic foods are not pasteurized). If some-thing is cooked or has been refrigerated at all times, then it should be fine. Really, you are more prone to food poisoning of all types during pregnancy, so be cautious in general of anything that's been sitting out. If any food is questionable, throw it out! Make sure all meat is well cooked. Sorry, no sushi or rare steaks allowed.

Food Safety Chart

Often	Occasionally	Never
Fruits	Caffeine	Undercooked meat or fish
Vegetables	Salmon	Old deli meat
Glasses of water (8)	Tuna	Alcohol
Prenatal vitamin	Catfish	Tilefish
Protein with each meal	Shrimp	Shark
Something green daily	Sea bass	Swordfish
Whole grain breads	Candy or junk	Unpasteurized milk or juice

Toxoplasmosis. Toxoplasmosis is a parasite that can live in cat feces. If it is contracted during pregnancy, then it can cause severe pregnancy complications. You should avoid handling cat litter or being in the room when the cat litter is being changed. You can still pet your cat and be in the same room as the cat litter as needed.

Sweeteners. Neither aspartame (Equal) or sucralose (Splenda) have been shown to cause malformations or pregnancy complications.

Exercise. Staying active helps you maintain your overall stamina, avoid excess weight gain, and decrease your risk for gestational diabetes. If you are not already active, we recommend that you start walking or swimming thirty minutes daily, at least five times a week. As you exercise, you want to maintain your heart rate at under 150 beats per minute. This is an exertion level of about six to seven (on a scale of one to ten). At this level, you should still be able to talk.

If you are already active with an exercise routine such as running or aerobics, you can usually continue with the modifications mentioned—keeping your heart rate under 150 and being able to talk. It is also a good idea to maintain your flexibility and strength. A prenatal yoga or Pilates class (or DVD) can help you maintain your core muscles to reduce the back pain associated with the middle of a pregnancy. Additionally, weight lifting should be limited to less than forty pounds. After fifteen weeks, exercises that involve lying flat on your back should be avoided.

You should avoid activities that have a risk of trauma such as basketball, hockey, or horseback riding. Scuba diving should be avoided due to a risk of fetal decompression sickness (the bends). If you are a competitive or professional athlete, you should meet with your doctor as soon as possible to modify your specific routine as appropriate. There is a lot that is not known about strenuous exercise in pregnancy. Most conditioned athletes are able to continue a modified version of their exercise routine, while some will develop signs that the baby is not growing appropriately. Your doctor will need to know the amount of exercise you are getting and can recommend appropriate testing.

These recommendations for exercise apply to healthy, uncomplicated pregnancies. If you have medical conditions or pregnancy complications, then your activity may need to be modified.

Warning signs that you should stop exercising:

- Chest pain or difficulty breathing
- Contractions
- Vaginal bleeding
- Dizziness
- Decreased fetal movement

Miscarriage

With advancing technology, women are finding out that they are pregnant much sooner than ever before. Early detection of pregnancy is sometimes good, but honestly it can also be a bad thing. Studies done using very sensitive blood tests have determined that up to thirty percent of pregnancies are "lost" before a woman's menstrual cycle. If the patient had not taken the pregnancy test, she would not have realized that she was pregnant. This type of loss is medically referred to as a "chemical pregnancy." I don't mean to minimize the pain associated with these early losses, but medically *miscarriage* is defined as a loss of a pregnancy between four and twenty weeks (loss after twenty weeks is referred to as a *stillbirth*).

Symptoms of a miscarriage include:

- Bleeding
- Spotting
- Cramping
- Pain

Sadly, miscarriage is very common. Before I go into those statistics, I want to start by telling you the positives.

- A healthy woman who is younger than thirty-two and is pregnant for the first time has a twelve percent risk of miscarriage.
- Her risk drops to eight percent after a yolk sac is seen on ultrasound (approximately five weeks).
- Her risk drops to three percent when a heartbeat is seen and the baby is one centimeter long (approximately seven weeks).
- So essentially, at her first doctor's appointment with a good heartbeat detected, her chances of having a healthy baby are ninety-seven percent.[3]

What if you don't fall into these categories? Then we need to consider the other main risk factor, which is age. For healthy women aged thirty-five to thirty-nine, the risk of miscarriage ranges from seventeen to thirty percent. For women

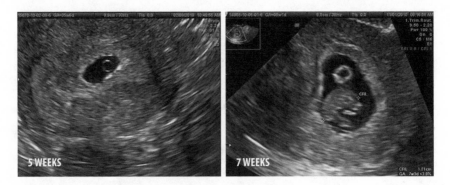

5 WEEKS   7 WEEKS

over the age of forty, the risk increases further, ranging from forty to fifty percent. We still see a decreased risk of loss after seeing a heartbeat (ten percent), but unfortunately, it is not as reassuring as in the younger patient.

If the patient experienced a miscarriage in her last pregnancy, the risk does goes up, but the risk is not additive. After one miscarriage, the risk goes up to twenty-four percent, but after two it is only twenty-six percent. After three losses, the risk is thirty-four percent. So even if you've had six miscarriages, your chance of having another is only fifty percent. If you have had children in between miscarriages, your odds of having a healthy pregnancy increase significantly.

Of course, the most common question associated with pregnancy loss is this: What causes miscarriage? There are several different factors that contribute. Some are treatable, but most are not. The most common cause is genetic abnormality. Between seventy-five and ninety percent of all miscarriages are caused by a genetic abnormality of the baby, meaning that the baby's chromosomes did not form properly. While it is discouraging that this is not preventable, it can also be encouraging that it's not recurrent. We also think this is why we see the increased risk of miscarriage with age. As we age, there is more damage to our DNA as it replicates. These errors are passed on to the embryo, and the result is abnormal chromosomes. The two most common genetic abnormalities found in miscarriages are Turner's syndrome and Down syndrome. So the majority of the time, the reason for miscarriage is unavoidable.

There is an increased risk of miscarriage in smokers, those who drink more than two alcoholic beverages per day, and heavy caffeine drinkers (greater than three cups of coffee daily). These behaviors can be modified to decrease your risk of miscarriage.

Despite what your girlfriend or your paranoid mother has told you, the following things do not cause miscarriage:

- Stress
- Lifting a box, or your toddler for that matter
- Having sex
- Exercise

So when should you be worried? After how many miscarriages? I once attended an infertility conference and watched the two most well-respected infertility specialists in the field debate this question for ten minutes. So if you read another "expert" give a different opinion on the matter, don't be surprised.

Recurrent miscarriage is usually defined as two losses without any live births or three total losses. So, after two or three miscarriages, most doctors recommend further testing. Other factors such as age and infertility history are taken into account as well in deciding when to offer testing. If you do have recurrent miscarriages, these are the tests routinely done to look for other modifiable medical causes.

Genetic. The patient and her partner are tested to confirm that they have normal chromosomes. This is a blood test called a karyotype.

Hormonal. A blood test checks for hormonal imbalances such as thyroid disorder, diabetes, and prolactinoma. Having poorly controlled diabetes can increase your risk for miscarriage.

Structure of the uterus. Your doctor checks to see if the actual womb is of normal shape. This can best be seen through a test called an HSG, which involves pushing dye through the uterus and taking an X-ray. This test may also be done as part of the workup for infertility (see Chapter One).

Immunologic. This blood test checks for antiphospholipid antibody syndrome. With this syndrome, the body can form a type of immune response to the pregnancy. This condition is rare and is usually associated with loss of a pregnancy in the second trimester.

Types of Miscarriage

Medically, we refer to miscarriages as "complete" versus "incomplete." This terminology has to do with whether the baby is still in the uterus or not. If the baby has completely passed and the uterus is empty, a woman has had a complete miscarriage. At this point, the doctor will normally just follow you up routinely.

If the tissue is still in the uterus, it is called an incomplete miscarriage. Here the doctor will advise you to wait until the tissue passes on its own, or she'll perform a D & C (dilation and curettage). This choice will depend on the size of the tissue and your personal desires. Waiting for the tissue to pass can take several weeks and can be emotionally challenging. Also at times the bleeding can become quite heavy, necessitating a D & C. If the tissue hasn't passed on its own after several weeks, then there is an increased chance of infection, so a D & C is recommended. A D & C is a minor surgery that removes the tissue. Your risk with this surgery is low, but all surgeries have a small chance of complications such as bleeding or infection.

D & C

Dilation and curettage is not abortion. I find some women resistant to a D & C because they think it is an abortion. This confusion is compounded by the fact that in medical lingo *all* pregnancy losses are referred to as abortions. This is just the medical term, but when people see that word on their medical forms, it can cause an emotional response at an already overly emotional time.

A D & C is a minor outpatient surgery that involves removing the lining and contents of the uterus. It is done for a variety of reasons, including postmenopausal bleeding, fibroids, miscarriage, and yes (by some) to terminate early pregnancies. It is important to understand that having a miscarriage that is medically treated by a D & C is in *no way* an abortion.

The Doctor's Point of View (POV): Miscarriage

In my first attempt to get pregnant, we conceived the first month. We were overjoyed, calling all our family immediately after the test was positive. We had waited eight years after getting married, so we had been planning this for a long time. The excitement was short-lived when after only a few days I began bleeding. We were devastated. The grief was profound, despite the loss coming so early. At first I regretted telling people so soon, but as I moved forward, I felt that it helped for people to know why I was sad. Many gave me their own words of encouragement from their loss experiences.

We tried again a few months later and conceived our oldest son. Things went well, and I delivered a healthy baby boy. The entire first trimester, though, I was filled with anxiety, as I waited to get to the "safety zone."

Now, in my practice, miscarriage is something I commonly have to treat. After experiencing one myself, I think it helps me have an extra layer of compassion and understanding for the level of loss involved.

The Patient's POV: Miscarriage

I took a break from writing this chapter when I experienced my third miscarriage. How's that for research? This time I had a heterotopic pregnancy, which means I conceived twins—one made it to my uterus but never fully formed, and the other implanted in my right tube, a part of my reproductive system which now, I'm sorry to say, is a distant memory. I share this so you will know that I really do understand where you are if you are experiencing or have experienced a miscarriage. It seems as though pregnancy loss is more and more common these days. That is in part due to early pregnancy detection, as we learned earlier in this chapter. I believe it is also due to the fact that we live in a fallen world where bad things just happen.

My first miscarriage occurred at around seven weeks and after we had heard a heartbeat. I experienced bleeding for about a week and then went on to pass the baby and all of the other parts present at this level of gestation. The bleeding lasted another week. The experience was painful both physically and emotionally, partly due to the fact that it all happened naturally and over time.

My second miscarriage was a bit different. We went in for our twelve-week ultrasound and discovered there was no longer a heartbeat. Our baby had died at around eight weeks, and we never knew it. Because my body had not yet begun the process of releasing the pregnancy, we decided to have a D & C, as I could not bear the thought of carrying the baby any longer. The D & C was not very invasive and allowed Dr. Rupe to perform a chromosomal analysis on the baby to determine that she had Turner's syndrome (one of the most common chromosomal abnormalities that leads to miscarriage). I went on to bleed for about a week, but the pain was minimal.

My recent ectopic pregnancy has been one of the most physically painful experiences I have ever had. Although the loss was hard and devastating, I am so thankful for God's protection and Dr. Rupe's very capable hands that performed my surgery. With each loss, I've tried to make sense of it. This time, though, I was much more quick to resolve in my heart that God is God, and he loves me even though he's allowed me to go through these losses.

Because we will rarely discover the true reason for a miscarriage, we are left to put our trust in the Lord to give us and the doctors wisdom in how to move forward. You must guard your heart and mind from wondering and worrying and instead find a healthy balance between letting go and understanding what your body needs to sustain a pregnancy. While I don't want you to obsess about what your body is or isn't doing, you know your body better than anyone. It helps to remain in tune with what is happening, as you may be able to guide the doctors in discovering what will work for you.

Common Questions You May Have This Month

I thought it was supposed to be "morning" sickness. Help! I'm sick all day!
Sorry. Morning sickness is in fact a misnomer. Although the nausea is often worse in the morning, it can occur all day long. Refer back to the tips in this chapter for keeping nausea to a minimum.

I've been training for a marathon, but I just found out I am pregnant. Can I run in the race?
It's really going to depend on your level of conditioning, but probably not unless you are an elite runner. (If you don't know what an elite runner is, then you are not one.) Though there has never been a report of exercise-induced heat malformation, talk with your doctor about your risk. It may be best to drop down to the half marathon or 5K.

Is it OK to have sex during pregnancy?
Yes. If it does not cause bleeding or pain, it is fine to have sex. If you develop risk complications such as preterm labor or placenta previa, your doctor may restrict your activities at that point.

Is it OK to get the flu shot during pregnancy? Some people say I should wait until after the first trimester. I'm confused.

Yes, it is safe to get the flu shot during pregnancy at any time. The previous recommendations were to wait until after twelve weeks; however, these guidelines changed about ten years ago. Some doctors still wait until after the first trimester to give the shot—not because it's not safe but because the average first trimester miscarriage rate is about fifteen percent. By waiting to get the flu shot, patients won't inappropriately blame the vaccine if something does go wrong. Please do note that the live virus nasal vaccine is not safe during pregnancy.

I have a really stressful job. Can that hurt my baby?

No. Emotional stress does not increase your risk of miscarriage. You do not need to "stress about your stress." Just relax and pray for peace for both your job *and* your pregnancy.

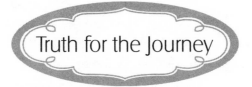
Truth for the Journey

Many, O Lord My God, are the wonders you have done. The
things you planned for us no one can recount to you; were
I to speak and tell of them, they would be too many to declare.
Psalms 40:5

At this point in your pregnancy, you are likely just trying to get used to the idea of being pregnant and all that it means to be expecting a child. Dr. Rupe addressed many details this month, most importantly pregnancy restrictions. After reading the list of things you should and shouldn't do, you might be wondering why you got yourself into this in the first place. While it's true that you have to make many adjustments in pregnancy, the major rules are pretty minor in the grand scheme of things. Still, it can be overwhelming to remember what you shouldn't eat, what medications you can take, or how fast your heart should beat during exercise.

That is why I want to focus right now on the wonder that is going on inside of you. We touched on this briefly last month, and we'll talk about it often in the book—and rightfully so. I don't think I will ever get tired of pondering the miracle and wonder of life. It's so much more enjoyable than pondering the rules and restrictions that come with being pregnant.

Many are the wonders God has done, including the one going on in you at this very moment. You may not truly connect to this reality until next month when you start to feel the baby move, but take a minute now to stop and think about the life growing inside you. Trust me when I tell you, that little person will be worth every adjustment you make over the next several months. This is only the beginning of the sacrifices you will make as a mother, but the love and the joy of raising a child will far outweigh the inconvenience of cutting down on caffeine for a few months.

Remember that exercise I asked you to do in the Introduction? You don't? No one ever reads the Introduction. Go back and read it now. There's some good stuff in there, including a great exercise to help you get rid of fears, frustrations, and overwhelming thoughts like what kind of fish you can have when you go out to dinner this weekend. OK, did you read it? Now take a deep breath. Let your heart and mind be filled with fresh faith, peace, and perspective. As you breathe out, let go of all of those overwhelming thoughts that want so badly to invade your mind. I know, I know, this idea is not new or mind-blowing, but it does help. After all, not only will it help clear your mind, but stopping to take deep and slow breaths can also help a queasy stomach. So breathe deep, my friend!

Journal everything during your pregnancy. You think you will always remember the little things, but you don't. The mind is not the same after pregnancy. Carrie, 36, mother of two

Instead of being overwhelmed by all of the new information that you have to absorb during pregnancy, I want you to remain focused with great expectation on the goodness and greatness of God. The God that so intricately created life and thought to bring it about in such an amazing way has got to be wonderful. Turn your heart and thoughts to him as you walk through these next seven or eight months, and I know you'll come to understand that wonder in a deep and intimate way.

We talked about miscarriage in this chapter, and I shared more of my story in the Patient's Point of View section. If you have experienced or think you are experiencing a miscarriage, my heart breaks for you. I understand your questions and your pain. Allow yourself time to grieve this loss. It may seem insignificant to some if miscarriage happens very early in the pregnancy. I am here to tell you there is nothing insignificant about the loss of a life, at any stage. Don't be afraid to be honest with God about your broken heart. He will come and cover you with his love.

Above all else, do not lose hope if you believe that you will have a child. Keep trusting God that he will prepare your body to carry the next pregnancy. He loves you and your mother's heart. After all, he created you for this great purpose. Be open to whatever story he's writing for you, but also be honest about the desires of your heart.

For some, maybe those with recurrent miscarriages or infertility, the pain may be deeper, so deep you may think you don't have the will to try again. Walk your journey one day at a time. Ask the Lord for just enough grace to get you through today, and then ask again tomorrow. As you walk with him daily, he will show you the next steps to take. Isaiah 30:21 says, "Whether you turn to the right or to the left, your ears will hear a voice behind you, saying, 'This is the way; walk in it.'" If you feel as though you want to give up, listen for his voice. He will show you when it's time to take another path. You may not be ready to consider "another path" right now and that is OK. As you continue to seek him and put your trust in him, he will align your heart with his will.

> During the first trimester, I always had a hard time believing I was pregnant. I didn't look pregnant, and I barely felt pregnant. After having several miscarriages, I struggled with fear immensely. One truth kept me strong . . . that God is the giver of life. The more I was able to trust him, the more peace I experienced. Kristy, 33, mother of three

Before we address other prayer concerns for this month, I want to stop now and include a prayer for those of you experiencing a miscarriage. If this doesn't include you, then I ask you to take a moment anyway and say your own prayer for those women who are experiencing a heart-breaking loss right now.

A Miscarriage Prayer

Oh Lord,

My heart is broken. I am disappointed and confused. My mind cannot comprehend why you would bring life to my body only to quickly take it away. But I know that your ways are higher than mine, and I must rest in that truth. I ask you to come now and cover me with your peace as I grieve this loss. Give me hope, Lord, that you will heal my body and my heart. Give me wisdom to know what steps to take next and give me strength to take them. I admit, Lord, that I do not understand your ways, but I trust your heart . . . and so I leave mine in your healing hands. Amen.

Prayer Concerns

Baby's development

Relief from "morning" sickness

Wisdom to follow guidelines

A Prayer for Your Journey

Dear Lord,

Many are the wonders you have done! I am honored to be a part of one of them. Thank you for the miracle you are creating within me. Please give me wisdom to make the right choices for my body and my baby. I ask you to give me strength as I adapt to life as a mommy-to-be. Thank you for continuing to develop my baby perfectly, according to your will. Amen.

Write a prayer here for your own personal journey.

_____

_____

_____

_____

_____

Journal

Record your thoughts and your fears here. It is important to acknowledge every thought and feeling you are experiencing. The main thing is to get them out in the open, and if they do not line up with the truth or the faith that you possess, then get rid of those burdens by giving them over to your Pregnancy Companion.

_____

_____

_____

_____

_____

Chapter Four

Keeping It Together
Weeks 11 to 15

Key Bible Verse

For by him all things were created: things in heaven and on earth, visible and invisible, whether thrones or powers or rulers or authorities; all things were created by him and for him. He is before all things, and in him all things hold together.

Colossians 1:16–17

Baby Stats

Your baby is 1½ inches long by eleven weeks and has progressed to the size of a large grape. Baby will declare itself boy or girl by twelve weeks and have fully defined legs by fifteen weeks. He's very active in the womb, though it is too early to feel movement (that is, of course, unless you have the world's most sensitive uterus). He weighs only a few ounces at this point, yet all the major organ systems are formed. By fifteen weeks, he's 3½ inches long, the size of a kiwi.

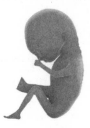

The good news is that the risk of miscarriage at this point is extremely low. Rejoice in the life that is within you!

Mommy Stats

Your uterus is beginning to grow. It is above your pubic bone by twelve weeks, expanding beyond your pelvis into your lower abdomen. If this is your first pregnancy, I am sorry to say it's most likely not baby if you are showing before twelve weeks. With future pregnancies, it does seem that women show earlier, which may be because their body remembers what it is supposed to do.

I once had a patient who had two successful pregnancies and then two miscarriages in a row. With her next pregnancy, she was a little anxious. At twelve weeks, she was concerned that she was still wearing her "regular" clothes. In her previous pregnancies, she had been in maternity clothes by this point. She confided her worries to her husband, who replied, "Don't worry honey, your regular clothes are just a lot bigger now than they used to be." Needless to say, that answer got him in the doghouse for a while. She went on to have a healthy baby girl.

All that to say, don't worry too much about how your body is showing at this point. Every woman is different and every one will carry differently. Just enjoy the fact that life is growing inside of you.

By this point, your blood volume has increased by fifteen percent, so if you've gained a pound or two, the blood is likely the culprit. Your body will increase its blood volume by 150 percent by the end of your pregnancy, so a lot of the weight you gain is fluid.

Symptom Checker

- ☐ Morning sickness
- ☐ Fatigue
- ☐ Frequent urination
- ☐ Constipation
- ☐ Heartburn
- ☐ Hunger (with cravings and aversions)
- ☐ Emotional instability
- ☐ Headaches
- ☐ Dizziness
- ☐ Occasional cramping

Your pregnancy hormone HCG level peaked at ten weeks, so as it decreases, your nausea and fatigue should begin to subside. This should make it easier to focus on getting a well-balanced diet and exercising four to five times per week. If you were too overwhelmed with fatigue to exercise in the first trimester, try again now. Remember that walking and swimming are two great exercise options for expectant mothers. Once again, make sure you are keeping your heart rate less than 150, which allows enough blood to flow to your uterus and baby.

You also want to avoid activities that put you at high risk for injury. Your coordination is going to be off due to your weight and body changes. Additionally, your joints are more lax due to pregnancy hormones, so you are prone to things like twisted ankles. If you've never done complex step aerobics, this wouldn't be the time to start. However, maintaining aerobic exercise is great for decreasing stress in pregnancy, reducing your risk for gestational diabetes, and keeping you strong for labor.

You may feel stretching and cramping during this phase, as your uterus begins to go places it's never gone before. If you notice cramping, make sure you are well hydrated and are having regular bowel movements. The uterus sits on the lower colon at this stage, so if you are constipated, it can make your uterus feel crampy. Constipation is a common symptom in pregnancy. Your body is always looking to stay hydrated, so it will draw all moisture out of the stools as they are passing through the colon. Increasing your fiber intake, drinking lots of water and, if necessary, taking a stool softener (like docusate sodium) can help maintain regular bowel movements, which will decrease cramping.

There are lots of strange pains and sensations during pregnancy, and it can be hard to know if those pains should be a concern to you or not. A good rule of thumb is that if a pain goes away with acetaminophen (Tylenol), hydration, and rest, it's not concerning. If it persists despite these measures, you should call your doctor.

Normal	Cause for Concern
Brief pains (< 1 minute)	Pain that gets worse even with rest
Cramps that resolve with rest and fluids	Pain with fever
Spotting after sex	Bleeding like period
Spotting after bowel movement	Spotting for no reason
Constipation	Diarrhea or vomiting (> 24 hours)

Symptoms that should cause concern are bleeding and severe pain. A small amount of spotting after intercourse or a pelvic exam is normal; anything beyond that should prompt an immediate call to your physician. By *spotting*, I mean streaks of blood (red or brown) on tissue with wiping or a very small amount on underwear. If you have vomiting or diarrhea for greater than twenty-four hours, you could be dehydrated and should seek medical attention.

Expectations for This Month's Visit

During your visit, your doctor will listen to the baby's heartbeat with the Doppler radar. If it takes her a few minutes to find the heartbeat, or she has to get out the ultrasound machine, don't be scared. Sometimes those little kiwis are hard to find in there.

She will also begin to discuss different options for screening for conditions such as Down syndrome and spina bifida in the baby. This is a very important topic and can be confusing, so I strongly encourage you to be prepared. Read this information thoroughly and really pray through this topic.

Doppler

The Doppler device uses ultrasound waves that travel through the maternal abdomen to detect the motion of the fetal heart. The ultrasound waves reflect off the fetal blood as it is pushed out of the heart and travel back to the sensor on the Doppler, giving the fetal heart rate. The fetal heartbeat cannot be heard by stethoscope until after twenty weeks of pregnancy, and even after twenty weeks, the Doppler still gives the heart rate more clearly. The fetal monitors in the hospital that record the fetal heart rate over time also use ultrasound Doppler technology.

Genetic Screening

I have a lot of patients who say to me as I begin to broach the subject of Down syndrome testing, "I'm a Christian. I would never have an abortion, so I don't want any genetic screening." Or they may say, "We'll love the baby no matter what, so it really doesn't matter to us." I've actually had people get mad at me for bringing up the topic. While these beliefs and feelings are valid, it is important to consider all the options.

Even if you would not choose to terminate the pregnancy, knowing about abnormalities can help you and your doctor plan for delivery. For instance, if the baby has Down syndrome (or any other type of syndrome), it is often helpful to deliver at a larger hospital with a neonatal specialist on staff. These babies can sometimes have special needs after delivery. Up to fifty percent of babies with Down syndrome will be born with a heart defect, so delivering at a hospital that has a pediatric cardiologist on staff would be beneficial. As another example, babies who have spina bifida are usually allergic to latex. If your doctor knew ahead of time, special precautions could be taken at the time of delivery. So, testing can have an effect on pregnancy management.

Down syndrome is caused when the baby has an extra twenty-first chromosome, and it is the most common genetic syndrome. The incidence for Down syndrome increases dramatically with the expectant mother's age. Here are the numbers:

At the age of 20, your risk of having a baby with Down syndrome is 1 in 2,000.
At the age of 35, your risk of having a baby with Down syndrome is 1 in 250.
At the age of 40, your risk of having a baby with Down syndrome is 1 in 69.
At the age of 45, your risk of having a baby with Down syndrome is 1 in 19.

Let's look at the numbers another way. What are your chances of having a baby that *does NOT* have Down syndrome?

At the age of 20, it is 99.95 percent.
At the age of 35, it is 99.6 percent.
At the age of 40, it is 98.6 percent.
At the age of 45, it is 94.8 percent.

Advanced Maternal Age

If you are pregnant and over age thirty-five, you are defined as having "advanced maternal age." Once again, thirty-five is not some terrible age where suddenly all babies have Down syndrome. It is important to note that being thirty-five or older does not make you "high risk" for all general pregnancy complications; however, age puts you in the higher risk category for genetic syndromes, which is an important thing to consider. If you look at total numbers, the majority of Down syndrome babies are actually born to women under the age of 35, because they have the majority of babies. I encourage you not to be fearful on your walk through pregnancy. God is the author of life, no matter what age the mother is!

The diagnostic testing options for Down syndrome include amniocentesis and chorionic villus sampling. Screening tests include nuchal translucency screening and the quad screen, which also screen for trisomy 18. Trisomy 18 is a more rare abnormality resulting in malformations that are not compatible with life. Current recommendations are to make all tests available to all patients and then to let them decide based on their age risk and their comfort level. Screening tests determine if you are at an increased risk, whereas diagnostic tests are used to confirm the diagnosis.

Amniocentesis

The amniocentesis was actually the first test developed for diagnosing genetic abnormalities. It involves inserting a needle into the amniotic fluid under ultrasound guidance, and it can be performed after sixteen weeks. The fluid is then extracted and sent for genetic testing. This test will tell you the exact genetic makeup of your baby. The main concern with this test is the risk of miscarriage. The risk of miscarriage from this test was originally 1 in 250. Current data shows the risk of miscarriage with amniocentesis to be lower, some centers with rates as low as 1 in 1,000.

Chorionic Villus Sampling

Another type of testing is chorionic villus sampling (CVS). This involves taking a small biopsy of the placenta by inserting a small tube through the cervix. A speculum is placed in the vagina, like when having a Pap smear. This test can be done between ten and fourteen weeks. The risk of miscarriage with this procedure is about 1 in 500. CVS is normally performed by a high-risk specialist.

Nuchal Translucency

The nuchal translucency screening is a specialized ultrasound that is performed between eleven and fourteen weeks. The ultrasound measures the thickness of the baby's neck. If the neck is abnormally thick, the test can indicate an increased risk for chromosomal anomalies (like Down syndrome and Turner's syndrome). Maternal blood is also drawn to check specific protein levels. The protein level and neck thickness are then put into an equation to determine the risk of abnormalities. This will detect Down syndrome about ninety percent of the time, but it is noninvasive and does not have a risk of miscarriage. There are false positives with this test (meaning that four percent of the time the test will show abnormal results, even though the baby is fine). So if the test is abnormal, you would be referred to a specialist for counseling to consider more definitive testing such as CVS or amniocentesis.

Quad Screen

The quad screen (previously called the *triple screen*) is a blood test that looks at maternal protein levels between sixteen and twenty weeks' gestation. If the protein levels are abnormal, it can indicate a chromosomal abnormality. This test will detect abnormalities eighty percent of the time. There are also false positives with this test. This test serves the same purpose as the nuchal screening but is available later in pregnancy.

Alpha-Fetoprotein

The alpha-fetoprotein (AFT) is a blood test that screens for spina bifida. Spina bifida is a structural problem, not a genetic one. Normally, the closure of the neural tube (where the spinal cord lives) occurs about twenty-eight days after fertilization. However, if something interferes and the tube fails to close properly, a neural tube defect will occur. Antiseizure medications, poorly-controlled diabetes, family history, obesity, and an increased body temperature from fever or external sources such as hot tubs can increase the chances a woman will carry a baby with spina bifida. Most women who give birth to babies with spina bifida have none of these risk factors. However, being on folic acid before conception can help prevent spina bifida. If your doctor knows ahead of time that the baby has spina bifida, special precautions can be taken at delivery to ensure the baby's safety.

I have definitely seen people regret getting tested. As I mentioned, there can be false positives. A small portion of the time, the tests will come back abnormal, but further testing will reveal that everything is OK with the baby. This is obviously very stressful for the family. At that point, they would have to decide whether or not to have an amniocentesis. Additionally, I have seen people who wished they had been tested. Sometimes later in pregnancy on ultrasound, we will see minor variations that can be associated with Down syndrome. This can make the expectant parents anxious, because tests (other than amniocentesis) are time sensitive and are not valid past twenty weeks' gestation.

Genetic testing is a very personal decision that you need to pray about. If you decide to decline testing, be prepared that some physicians will really push you to reconsider. It is your choice, though, so stick to your guns about what you feel is right. The reason many physicians will push for you to have testing is, sadly, because this issue is one over which many doctors get sued. There have been many cases of babies born with Down syndrome in which the patients sued the doctor because they weren't given the option for testing and abortion. So if you are asked to sign a consent form to decline testing, don't be offended.

Test	Screens	Accuracy	Timing	Risks to Baby
Nuchal translucency	– Down syndrome – Trisomy 18	85 percent	11–14 weeks	None
Quad screen	– Down syndrome – Trisomy 18 / 21 – Spina bifida	80 percent	15–20 weeks	None
Amniocentesis	– Chromosomal abnormalities (such as Down, etc.)	100 percent	After 15 weeks	Miscarriage rate 1 percent
Chorionic villus sampling	– Chromosomal abnormalities (such as Down, etc.)	100 percent	10–12 weeks	Miscarriage rate 1 percent

As you make the decision whether or not to have tests performed, consider your risk, your level of anxiety, and how you feel God is guiding you. If you are in your early twenties and struggle with fear in your life, then having these tests may not be the best idea for you. Your odds of having a baby with Down syndrome are very low, and if your test came back with a false positive, it could really be a struggle for you. However, if you are in your forties and you know your risk is high, it could be reassuring to know everything is OK.

The Doctor's POV: Genetic Screening*

When I had my son, the nuchal screen was not yet available. (I'm not that old—it's just a newer test!) I was twenty-seven at the time, so I knew my risk was relatively low. The quad screen has a higher rate of false positives (the test results are abnormal, but the test is wrong), and it seemed that many of my patients would get all worked up over an abnormal result, yet everything would be fine in the end. So after careful, prayerful consideration, we elected not to have any testing.

Our baby (we didn't know what we were having) developed dilated kidneys on ultrasound later in pregnancy. Dilated kidneys can be what is called a soft marker for Down syndrome. Soft markers are found in three percent of normal pregnancies (see page 102). I think sometimes when you know *all* the crazy things that can go wrong in pregnancy, it is challenging to not walk in fear. So there was a time when I did regret not having the test, because if the quad screen had been normal, then there would have been less to worry about with the dilated kidneys. Intellectually, I knew the odds were that the baby would be fine, but it was still hard not to worry.

After delivery, our son did great. His kidneys required close follow-up for a couple of years, but they now function normally, and he never needed surgery.

*I want to clarify that this was only my feeling as a patient when I was pregnant, not my medical opinion for others.

The Patient's POV: Genetic Screening

After experiencing my first two miscarriages, one as a result of a chromosomal abnormality, my husband and I went into our third pregnancy knowing that we wanted genetic testing done. Our belief was that although we trusted the Lord with this life, we would rather be prepared and not completely surprised like we were the last time.

The time came for my twelve-week visit where the ultrasound technician would perform the nuchal transluency test. We prayed and prayed, believing that everything would be normal but knowing that God might have other plans. We hoped for a good report, but we had to be ready for anything. We believed he was sustaining our baby because he is able and he is faithful, yet we also knew that sometimes he allows horrible things to happen because we live in a broken world. We just trusted that God would use those things for his glory—somehow.

As the technician performed the test, our squirmy little kiwi would not cooperate. She just wasn't in a position that would allow the tech or Dr. Rupe to see what they needed to see. I was definitely disappointed that I would not receive a good report that day, but I was also relieved that I wouldn't be receiving a bad one, either. Dr. Rupe explained the other testing options so that Dave and I could prayerfully consider them.

A few days later, I called Dr. Rupe to let her know we wouldn't be going through with any further testing. After much prayer and talking it through, Dave and I decided that the unsuccessful nuchal test was God's way of telling us to let it go. We didn't need to know what was going on in there. That was for him to be concerned with.

I clung tightly to Colossians 1:16–17, believing that he was holding my little one together. Dr. Rupe would get to check the baby's development during my twenty-week ultrasound, and we knew many issues could be detected then. That was all we needed to know to be at peace.

Six months later, I gave birth to a healthy baby girl, and honestly I breathed a huge sigh of relief. I would never recommend whether or not you should receive genetic testing. I just want to encourage you to be open to what God is saying about this topic. This is not merely about the testing; it's about the journey of faith you are on.

Common Questions You May Have This Month

I've developed varicose veins! Will they go away after I deliver?

Varicose veins usually increase in size during pregnancy. The more you stand, the worse they get. Compression stockings can help relieve some of the discomfort they cause. Some women also develop varicosities in their labia. All types of varicosity usually shrink significantly after birth, but they may not go away completely.

How do I prevent hemorrhoids?

There is no way to prevent hemorrhoids from forming. They are varicose veins of the rectum that tend to worsen during pregnancy and with pushing during delivery. Keeping constipation at bay with a high-fiber diet and staying well hydrated is your best bet for preventing them from getting worse.

I keep getting yeast infections! What's wrong?

First, you want your doctor to confirm that it really is a yeast infection. The usual symptoms are a cottage cheese type discharge, itching, and burning. They do seem to occur more often in pregnancy due to your decreased immune system as well as the increased discharge associated with pregnancy. Taking over-the-counter topical yeast medicine is safe in pregnancy. Increasing your yogurt intake can help keep your vaginal bacteria balanced. Be sure to avoid spending excess time in moist clothing like swimsuits or workout gear.

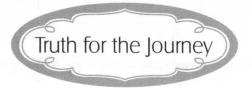

Truth for the Journey

For by him all things were created: things in heaven and on earth, visible and
invisible, whether thrones or powers or rulers or authorities; all things were created
by him and for him. He is before all things, and in him all things hold together.
Colossians 1:16–17

If I were a bettin' girl, I'd bet you are wondering about whether or not you should be showing by this point. Don't deny it. We've all been there. No matter how you size yourself up on a normal day, any day during your first trimester of pregnancy can make you feel completely abnormal and bloated. "Is this tummy pooch the baby, or did I eat too many fries? Gosh, fries taste so good to me right now!" As Dr. Rupe explained, if you think you are showing at this point, it's probably not baby. However, if you are like me—everything you put in your mouth goes straight to your belly—then exhale, my friend! No one really knows when you should or shouldn't be showing, so don't give it too much thought. Even some of the skinniest girls have little pooch bellies toward the end of their first trimester. Pretty soon, it's all going to catch up with you, and no one is going to remember if they began noticing your belly at twelve weeks or sixteen weeks. However, like Dr. Rupe said, it's so important to stay healthy during your pregnancy. So for goodness' sake, lay off the fries, will ya?

If you are really struggling with how you look or feel about yourself, that is completely normal. I encourage you to share your frustrations with your spouse or support system. Most importantly, share those thoughts with the Lord, and ask him to show you the truth about your beauty. There is nothing more beautiful than the miracle of life, and you are walking proof of that beauty right now. It may help to do something to pamper yourself, like taking a bubble bath (not too hot) or giving yourself a pedicure. Just remember that this is all part of the journey. Try to allow all of the bumps and curves in the road (and by bumps and curves I mean frustrations and feelings) to bring you closer to God and those around you. Being honest with yourself, the Lord, and your support system is the best way to accomplish this.

Savor the now. I spent my first pregnancy waiting for the arrival. If I could just take half of the worry I invested into it and instead focus on relishing the details of the pregnancy, I know I'd be the richer for it. Adrienne, 31, mother of two

You may have already shared your great news with friends and family, or perhaps you've been keeping it under wraps until you reach your second trimester. Each expectant mother may choose to handle this important announcement very differently. As you consider when and how to spread the word, you may deal with questions and bouts of fear, such as, "What if I tell too early and then have complications? My friend told too soon and then had a miscarriage. It was horrible." Or you might be thinking, "Is it wrong that I want to keep this precious news to myself for a while? I'm not in a hurry to receive all that unsolicited advice!" Each of these questions is very valid and very personal. Try not to look too closely at how others have handled their news. This is between you and God. This decision alone may bring you face-to-face with your biggest pregnancy fears, so lean into your Pregnancy Companion as you consider all of your options.

With each one of my pregnancies, my husband and I felt led to share the news with our friends pretty early on, partly because each of them had been believing with us for conception and partly because we needed the support to have faith through the early days of the pregnancy. Although it was hard to send the e-mail and make the calls with our first two miscarriages, it would have been much harder to suffer through them alone. Each and every person will feel differently about her situation. The simple solution is to tell when you feel led to tell.

It is normal to be concerned about the health of your baby, but we are reminded in the Bible that God is the author and sustainer of life. You must hold on to this truth throughout your pregnancy . . . especially now as you consider genetic testing. In this month's key Bible verse, Colossians 1:16–17, it says all things were created by God and in him all things hold together. He's created your unborn child, and God is presently and perfectly holding that child together with his great hands. Wow. If that doesn't make you feel a rush of peace, I'm not sure what will. This verse is the one I recited daily as I waited through my pregnancy.

I declared that God was holding together my little one and that his capable hand would deliver her to me perfectly formed and at the appointed time.

Meditate on the words of this passage as you pray through the important decision of genetic testing. Don't feel guilty if you feel led to have the testing done. Like Dr. Rupe mentioned, doctors can utilize the information no matter what the results are. The important thing is that you are led by the Lord and in agreement with your spouse or support system.

If you have genetic testing done and the results are concerning, don't panic. Discuss the results with your doctor and ask questions. Above all else, continue to pray and ask God to protect your baby's development. I pray this verse over you while you wait and trust God: "May the God of hope fill you with all joy and peace as you trust in him, so that you may overflow with hope by the power of the Holy Spirit" (Rom. 15:13). As you continue to deal with all of the questions and emotions that come with your first trimester nearing its end, remember that he holds things together in his capable hands.

Prayer Concerns

Baby's growth and development
Mommy's health
Dealing with the way you look
Deciding when to share the news
Genetic testing

A Prayer for This Month

Dear Lord,

I know my baby's life is in your hands—the same hands that so intricately created it. Help me to be led by your Spirit as I consider every option for this pregnancy, genetic testing most of all. I do not want to walk in fear, Lord. I trust you to develop my baby according to your divine purpose. Lead me and guide me as I consider this testing. Help me also, Lord, to see myself the way you see me as my body begins to change. Guard me against vanity and obsession regarding my pregnant body. I believe you are good and sovereign, and I thank you for this life. May your will be done. In Jesus' name, amen.

Write a prayer here for your own personal journey.

_____

_____

_____

_____

_____

Journal

Record your thoughts and your fears here. It is important to acknowledge every thought and feeling you are experiencing. The main thing is to get them out in the open, and if they do not line up with the truth or the faith that you possess, then get rid of those burdens by giving them over to your Pregnancy Companion.

_____

_____

_____

_____

_____

Chapter Five

What's Going On in There?
Weeks 16 to 20

Key Bible Verse

For you created my inmost being; you knit me together in my mother's womb. I praise you because I am fearfully and wonderfully made; your works are wonderful, I know that full well. My frame was not hidden from you when I was made in the secret place. When I was woven together in the depths of the earth, your eyes saw my unformed body. All the days ordained for me were written in your book before one of them came to be.

Psalms 139:13–16

Baby Stats

At twenty weeks, your baby is up to 6 ½ inches in length and weighs just under a pound. His head is still disproportionately bigger than his body, but his arms and legs are growing and catching up. By twenty weeks, he assumes the fetal position, as he is too big to fully stretch out. Baby's skin is developing, and he has his own distinct fingerprints that will belong to him forever.

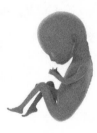

Mommy Stats

At this point in pregnancy, most women feel pretty good. Your HCG levels have begun to drop and your energy level is picking back up. Your body is adjusting to pregnancy. Depending on your height and build, you may or may not be "showing"; however, by now you will most likely need maternity pants. Even if you don't have a significant belly bump, your clothes probably feel a bit snug. By twenty weeks, the top of your uterus should be to your belly button.

This can be a time where anxiety begins to set in because you feel good. You no longer have the nausea to remind you that you are pregnant, but it's also usually too early to feel fetal movement. Even though you may not feel pregnant, rest assured you are at very low risk of miscarriage at this point in pregnancy.

After twenty weeks, try to sleep on your side and not flat on your back. As I mentioned, your baby-filled uterus reaches your belly button by twenty weeks. If you sleep flat on your back, your uterus lies on top of your aorta and vena cava, which are the main blood supply to and from your heart from the lower part of your body. A decreased blood flow here can make you feel dizzy and decrease the blood going to the uterus. It's best to sleep on your side, but if it doesn't work for you, at least put pillows under one side of your back, so that you are tilted and not flat.

Let me tell you, despite what other books may say, *it does not matter what side you sleep on!* In rare instances, women with high-risk pregnancies will be instructed to lie mainly on their left side, as this maximizes the blood flow to the uterus. For the average pregnant woman, however, it does not matter which side she lies on. It is difficult enough at the end of pregnancy to find a comfortable sleeping position, so limiting you to just one side is unnecessary. Most women do not have issues sleeping at this point, but if you do, you might consider a body pillow. I have many patients who love the huge, "C" shaped body pillows. They can reduce the hip discomfort that comes with sleeping on your side.

Symptom Checker

☐ Constipation

☐ Heartburn

☐ Hunger (with cravings and aversions)

☐ Emotional instability

☐ Headaches

☐ Dizziness

☐ Cramping

☐ Ligament pain

☐ Increased vaginal discharge

☐ Back pain

☐ Swelling

☐ Stomach flutter

Round ligament pain. Often around eighteen weeks, women will begin to experience ligament pain. The round ligament is a support structure that attaches from your uterus to your abdominal wall and then travels through your groin to attach to your pubic bone. As your uterus grows, this ligament begins to grow and stretch in ways it has never stretched before. This causes a sharp pain that radiates to your groin and usually gets better when you rest. It may also occur when you twist at the waist or roll over in bed. For most women, the pain is mild and can be managed with rest. If you are on your feet a lot for your job, then you may need a pregnancy support belt, which is basically a bra for your pregnant belly. The belt will help take some of the pressure off your hips and ligaments. You can find them at medical supply stores.

How do you know it's ligament pain? If the pain resolves with rest, it is most likely ligament pain and not worrisome. If there is numbness, weakness, or bleeding, then you should contact your doctor because it may be something else.

Vaginal discharge. Your uterus is growing exponentially at this point. It is already twenty times bigger than it was before baby took up residence there. Your cervix, the bottom part of your uterus, is growing and changing as well. It's what opens up to let the baby come out. The cervix sits at the top of the vagina, and its glands produce your vaginal discharge, which will become more copious and thick during pregnancy. Reasons to be concerned about vaginal discharge include itching, pain, strong odor, and change in color (white, clear, or light yellow is normal). If you experience these symptoms, check with your doctor because you could have a yeast or bacterial infection. If you have more discharge than usual but no other symptoms, it's perfectly normal.

Expectations for This Month's Visit

Your visit will more than likely include an anatomy ultrasound, which is routinely done in pregnancies between eighteen and twenty weeks. In low-risk pregnancies, it may be the last ultrasound performed. During this ultrasound, the technician checks a long list of things to make sure baby is growing appropriately. It can sometimes take a long time (up to forty minutes) for the technician to measure all the different structures on her list, especially if baby is being uncooperative with his position.

I've often had patients remark on how nervous they get during the ultrasound. They worry because it takes so long, and that must mean there is something wrong. I've also had patients express concern about the look on the technician's face as he or she performs the ultrasound. These perceptions, coupled with the fact that most technicians are instructed not to tell the patients any specifics, can indeed lead to anxiety for an unprepared patient. Simply remember going in that it is normal for this ultrasound to take awhile and for the technician's face to show frustration because he or she has to concentrate so hard on the monitor.

Believe it or not, the sole purpose of the anatomy ultrasound is not to find out the sex of your baby. The main areas of focus are the heart and the brain. Your technician will carefully inspect each heart valve to see if the blood is flowing properly and confirm that each tiny section of the brain is growing just right. Certain fluid collections around the brain can be a sign that the baby has spina bifida or other problems. If one of these problems is found, you should be referred to a specialist for further testing with more specialized ultrasound or MRI. While the idea of a heart defect is scary, knowing ahead of time can help the delivery team prepare to take the best possible care of baby after he is born. If it happens to be a rare defect, you may need to deliver at a larger hospital so the baby can be cared for by a specialist.

If the technician is not able to see all the structures on her list, you will be asked to come back in a couple of weeks for another view. Being overweight is one factor that can make it difficult for the technician to see the baby. The thicker the abdominal wall, the more difficult it is to see the baby. For some overweight women, despite multiple ultrasounds, we are never able to get the views we need of certain organs. This does not necessarily mean anything is wrong, it just means that they couldn't see all the parts that they needed to see.

Common Soft Markers

Soft markers are *not* physical abnormalities of the baby but rather a set of unusual ultrasound findings. They represent things seen on ultrasound that are not necessarily normal but are not considered malformations. Remember, ultrasound is a black-and-white, two-dimensional picture. So some of these markers are just things that show up as a brighter shade of white than normal. With the improvement in ultrasound technology, we began to discover these soft markers commonly in babies that had Down syndrome. The catch is that up to three percent of normal pregnancies also have these findings. Therefore, the following soft markers can lead to a lot of stress if you don't understand the significance (or lack thereof) of the findings.

Echogenic focus. *Echogenic* in ultrasound language means "bright" or "white." So an echogenic focus is just that, a very bright area on the ultrasound picture of the heart. The actual valves have increased mineral deposits in them. They are shaped normally and function normally. This finding does not reflect heart disease in any way. Many physicians believe echogenic foci to be normal variant.

Echogenic bowel. An echogenic bowel is just a very bright area on the bowel. This does not reflect any abnormal bowel function. This can be associated with cystic fibrosis, which can be tested easily during a pregnancy by a blood test on the mother. If echogenic bowel is present,the risk of Down syndrome is doubled. So if you are 35, and your ultrasound shows echogenic bowel then your risk goes from 1:250 to 1:125; which is still a less than 1% chance.

Choroid plexus cyst. This is a small cyst within the brain, though it may be better to think of it as a "fluid collection." The brain has the consistency of a sponge. As it grows and develops, it has to expand to fill the entire head. The choroid plexus cyst represents an area that the sponge hasn't fully expanded to fill. The cyst normally resolves by twenty-eight weeks. This is not associated with any brain abnormality or any kind of mental defect. If the cysts are located on both sides of the brain and do not resolve, then the risk of trisomy 18 is doubled.

Dilation of fetal kidneys. This is a swelling of the tube (the ureter) that connects the kidney and the bladder. While the swelling is technically a structural issue, it will resolve on its own most of the time. Babies born with this condition will need ultrasounds of their kidneys during the first year of life. If the swelling is on both kidneys then the risk of Down syndrome is doubled. Occasionally they will need surgery to correct it, but that is very rare.

About three percent of women will have one of these soft markers on their anatomy ultrasound. I try to explain to my patients the significance or lack thereof in these findings. If they have not yet had testing for genetic screening, I will usually recommend it to give them peace of mind. If the baby has three or four soft markers, then the risk of chromosomal abnormality (such as Down syndrome or trisomy 18) is further increased. In these instances, the patient may need to see a geneticist and consider further genetic testing. Usually the next test to confirm any diagnosis would be an amniocentesis.

On the flip side, fifty percent of Down syndrome babies have normal ultrasounds. So the majority of pregnancies that have abnormal ultrasounds (contain "soft markers") are actually fine, but up to half of pregnancies with Down syndrome babies have normal ultrasounds. While ultrasound is an amazing tool for the obstetrician in so many ways, it is not meant to "diagnose Down syndrome," despite common misconceptions.

The technology behind ultrasound has come a long way. We can find heart defects and other structural issues that can help us better prepare for the baby's birth. We can make sure growth is appropriate. We can make sure the placenta is in the correct position and look for signs of preterm labor. Most importantly, it gives us cute baby pictures to put as our screen saver.

Doctor's POV: It's a ??!!

"Are you going to find out what you're having?" is often one of the first questions people will ask when they find out you are pregnant. Medically, there's usually not a reason to find out, but in my practice I would say at least ninety-five percent of people learn the sex at their twenty-week ultrasound. My husband and I chose to keep it a surprise, much to the chagrin of our friends and family. As an obstetrician, I always enjoy the suspense of those deliveries where the sex is unknown. When I get to shout "It's a girl!" and hear the cheers go up around the delivery room, it's the best feeling. It really drove my mom crazy (this was her first grandchild) that we didn't find out. We had many conversations that went like this.

"So, you are really not going to find out?"

"NO."

"And you have an ultrasound in your office . . . that you know how to use . . . "

"Yes."

"SO you could look at any moment?"

"Yes."

"And you don't?"

"No."

"WHY?!"

I did have trouble finding a unisex nursery design at first and almost wavered in my decision, but I finally I found one I liked, so we were good to wait. We had also picked out a unisex name (Ryan). With so much modern technology available, to me it was fun to do something the old-fashioned way.

Oh yeah, and by the way, it was a BOY!

The Patient's POV: It's a ??!!

I always knew I would find out the sex of our baby. I am a planner, and knowing what we were having would allow me to plan accordingly. I'd been dreaming about baby names for years before I actually conceived, so the sooner I could name that little peanut, the better. We were able to find out what we were having pretty early on. My husband and I were sure it would be a boy. We both just had a feeling. At fifteen weeks, we went in for an ultrasound, and they were able to see that we were having a girl. Because it was so early, they weren't completely sure, but they were sure enough for me to start picking out pink paint. We were wrong with our prediction, but we were not disappointed in the least. Now I cannot imagine my life without princesses and dress-up clothes.

Finding out what we were having allowed us to bond early on with the life that was growing inside me. We gave her a name that we'd prayed about for months, and we began to dream about what her little personality would be like.

Whatever you decide to do in regard to finding out the sex of your baby will be the right choice for you. You may find it much more exciting to be surprised on delivery day when the doctor announces, "It's a ??!!" This is simply one of those decisions that is completely personal and never wrong no matter what you decide.

Common Questions You May Have This Month

Can you have too many ultrasounds?
We're not sure. There is a small amount of radiation associated with ultrasound; however, there has never been a single case of any type of abnormality linked to multiple ultrasounds. The current recommendation is that ultrasounds be done when they are medically necessary.

Should I get one of those 3D/4D ultrasounds?
I think that if you look at 3D ultrasounds solely as entertainment and don't get them often, then yes, having one should be fine. Now, I will give you this caveat. When I was pregnant, I had one done, and my baby looked really terrible! The baby is in very close quarters and often his hands or feet (or both) are pushing against his face, contorting it in crazy ways. So don't freak out if your baby looks weird in any ultrasound. I can assure you that in real life he will be adorable.

I know the recommendation is that ultrasound be used only when medically necessary, but experts also say that there has never been a case of harm known to be caused by ultrasound. So while you shouldn't have an ultrasound every day, getting an extra one to see how cute your little guy is should be fine.

Can I go to rock concerts or car races when I'm pregnant? Will the noise hurt my baby?
The noise is not going to hurt your baby. Your baby is floating in amniotic fluid, which will muffle any noise. I would caution you, though, against the mosh pit or crowd surfing while pregnant.

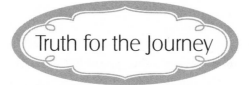

Truth for the Journey

For you created my inmost being; you knit me together in my mother's womb. I praise you because I am fearfully and wonderfully made; your works are wonderful, I know that full well. My frame was not hidden from you when I was made in the secret place. When I was woven together in the depths of the earth, your eyes saw my unformed body. All the days ordained for me were written in your book before one of them came to be.
Psalms 139:13–16

It can make you absolutely crazy not knowing what's going on in there. If you prefer to be in control like me, you probably spend countless hours wondering and trying to figure out what every twinge and pain means. It may seem like I am repeating myself in each chapter on the subject of worry versus peace of mind. It may seem like it because I am. Peace of mind is the most important heart issue that you will deal with during pregnancy. We all worry to some extent during our nine or ten months of baby growth and development. It's best to get a handle on it now so that you can begin to focus on other things in the weeks to come.

Practical Ways to Fight Fear, Anxiety, and Worry

1. Memorize scripture.
2. Stop whatever you are doing and breathe, then pray.
3. Write a prayer of declaration.
4. Talk with someone about your concerns.

I want to share with you a story from a time in my pregnancy when God pretty much whipped my butt into shape regarding worry. Actually, it's a funny story, which shows you that God cares enough about our thoughts and our peace of mind to lovingly and laughingly discipline us from time to time.

Keep in mind my first two pregnancies did not make it past twelve weeks. After two miscarriages, I was understandably on guard when it came to anything out of the ordinary. I was nineteen weeks pregnant, and we were getting ready for church one Sunday morning, when suddenly I sneezed. This was a big ole sneeze, and as I let it out, something abnormal happened. I felt a little fluid down below, so I did what any post-miscarriage, nineteen-week-pregnant mom-to-be would do—I referred to my pregnancy bible. "If you feel leaking fluid," the book explained, "you may have broken or punctured your amniotic sac. Call your doctor immediately." I put the book down and dialed Dr. Rupe's office. Since it was a Sunday, I received a return phone call from one of Dr. Rupe's colleagues. I explained what had happened and that I wondered whether I was leaking amniotic fluid. She obviously didn't know my history when she candidly replied, "If you are, then there's nothing we can do to save the baby at this point. But come in to the ER so we can check you out."

You can imagine my tension level while driving twenty minutes to the emergency room. My husband and I didn't say one word to each other, but we both knew that we were thinking the same things. We arrived at the ER, and they completed an ultrasound. To our delight, they discovered that everything was fine with our baby and my amniotic sac. In fact, I had merely peed in my pants upon sneezing, an embarrassing side effect for many expectant moms. I've never been more excited to have peed in my pants in my life! We laughed the entire way home, and I knew the Lord was smiling down on me, saying, "Why can't you just trust me?"

We're talking a lot about fear and anxiety during this chapter because, even though you are almost beyond the miscarriage zone, you are likely still awaiting the BIG ultrasound that checks out baby's organs and growth. I remember feeling like I was holding my breath until after that ultrasound. Those feelings are completely normal, but they do not have to overtake your heart and mind. If you receive a worrisome report after your ultrasound, I encourage you to remain calm and talk to your doctor thoroughly about the results. Feelings of worry and fear are to be expected, but remember that God can bring peace in the midst of this storm. The best thing you can do is to pray and lean into your family and friends for support as you wait for more conclusive information.

Read the verses in Psalm 139 again. Actually, if you have the time, read the entire chapter. What an amazing reminder of how the Lord intimately knows and cares for us. What an awesome picture of how he is knitting your child together, right now. He knows every cell and every hair. He's formed every finger and every toe. He ordained this life even before you conceived. Will you trust him with it?

Choosing a Baby Name

Choosing your baby's name might be one of the most fun aspects of expecting. There are many books and websites out there to help you choose a baby name, and several even give scriptures and Christian meanings for baby names. Perhaps you have decided to wait until your little one graces the world before you choose a name. This is an exciting way to welcome baby. I hope it hits you clearly when you see baby's sweet face what his or her name should be. If you are a planner like me, you probably have a list of names and middle names that you've been pining over for months.

Either way, I encourage you to pray about what to name your child. I love the idea of choosing a name with a strong and relevant meaning for each unique child. It's fine, too, if you'd rather just pick something cute with a good ring to it and don't really care about what the name means. As with many other choices you will make as a parent, there is no right or wrong here. It's simply up to you. Be careful though not to get too trendy, or your child may be disappointed later in life.

> When you are pregnant, *enjoy* your regular time with God, and when your baby arrives, make sure you have a *new* strategy set in place for it in this season, so you can be fueled and ready for parenting each day! Angela, 32, mother of two

Spending time with God each day may already be challenging for you. Let's face it: life gets busy, and sometimes our quiet time is the first thing to go when other things vie for our attention. Perhaps you've found a good rhythm of meeting with the Lord daily, and your time with him is regular. Whatever the case, once you welcome your baby into your home, there will be a real-life, legitimate little person begging for your attention for what seems like every minute of every day. As hard as it might be to find time to spend with the Lord in this new season, doing so will be the best thing you can do for yourself and your family.

Ask God to show you new strategies for spending time with him. When my daughter was an infant, I would come downstairs every morning when it was time to start the day, and I would feed her while reading the Bible aloud to her. Of course I knew she couldn't understand one word of it, but there was something so powerful about speaking God's Word over my child. I felt like I was doing something meaningful for her while fueling myself for another day. It is important to remember that the method you use to spend time with God may change as your child grows older. Be open to his leading. Simply bring your honest and longing heart before him, and he will meet you where you are.

Prayer Concerns

Baby's growth and development
Mommy's health
Ultrasound findings
Peace of mind

A Prayer for This Month

Dear Lord,

I am so glad that you know what's going on in there! Help me to trust that you are knitting my baby together with your very capable hands. I pray for great peace as we have our big ultrasound. Lord, help us to trust you no matter what the findings. Guide the doctors and technicians to see only what you need them to see. Protect us against any unnecessary concern. Thank you that our child is being fearfully and wonderfully made. Amen.

Write a prayer here for your own personal journey.

Journal

Record your thoughts and your fears here. It is important to acknowledge every thought and feeling you are experiencing. The main thing is to get them out in the open, and if they do not line up with the truth or the faith that you possess, then get rid of those burdens by giving them over to your Pregnancy Companion.

_____

_____

_____

_____

_____

Chapter Six

Now Showing . . . My Belly
Weeks 21 to 25

Key Bible Verse

If you remain in me and my words remain in you, ask whatever you wish, and it will be given you. This is to my Father's glory, that you bear much fruit, showing yourselves to be my disciples.
John 15:7–8

Baby Stats

Your baby is fully formed by twenty-four weeks, but he still needs some development. He is twelve inches in length (crown to heel) and weighs in at around 1½ pounds. By twenty-three weeks, the baby can hear sounds inside the womb. His eyes will begin to open at times. He's moving a lot, so his position is constantly changing. He may be head down one day and feet down the next. Many of my patients are concerned when their baby is breech at this point in pregnancy. I try to reassure them that baby's position now is unrelated to his position at term.

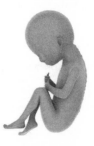

Babies born after twenty-four weeks have the potential to survive on their own. This potential is referred to as *viability*. A baby born at this stage, however, is an extreme preemie. He requires extended time in the neonatal intensive care unit (NICU) and needs help breathing for some time after birth. When babies born this early survive, they often have various challenges, including learning disabilities, breathing problems, and damage to their vision. Outcomes improve significantly with each passing week that the baby spends in the uterus, and by thirty-two weeks, most babies survive with no long-term issues.

While knowing that the baby could live if delivered may be reassuring, you definitely don't want to deliver just yet. Around this time, people love to tell you horror stories about preterm deliveries. I have no idea why people try to scare pregnant women. They just aren't thinking about how such stories could keep you awake at night. Rest assured, you have a low risk of having one of these stories of your own. See Chapter Ten for the facts about preterm births. The average, healthy, first-time mom has a ninety percent chance of a term delivery and a ninety-nine percent chance of delivering after thirty-two weeks.

Mommy Stats

Most moms will have a baby bump at this point, except for the tallest of moms. Remember that each woman carries her baby differently, so try not to compare yourself to your sister or neighbor or co-worker. More importantly, don't let it bother you when *other* people compare you to those people. If you have concerns about the size of your belly, bring it up with your doctor, but don't let random people in the elevator who ask if you are carrying twins get you down.

A woman of average weight should have gained about ten pounds at this point. The majority of this weight is fluid, both amniotic fluid and increased blood volume.

You should be feeling the baby move, but not necessarily every day. There is probably a lot of variation in the amount of movement you feel. Some days he may move like crazy, and other days you won't feel it at all. Baby's movements become more predictable at around twenty-eight weeks, so we will discuss movement-counting more in the next chapter. One thing that can affect your perception of movement is the location of the placenta. If the placenta is attached to the front of your uterus, you may not feel movement as strongly. The placenta acts as a cushion between you and the baby. So women with a placenta in the front of the uterus may not feel the movement until later in pregnancy—and may never feel them as strongly. Also, if you are overweight, you may not feel the movements as early.

Symptom Checker

- ☐ Constipation or hemorrhoids
- ☐ Heartburn
- ☐ Hunger (with cravings and aversions)
- ☐ Emotional instability
- ☐ Headaches
- ☐ Dizziness
- ☐ Cramping
- ☐ Ligament pain
- ☐ Increased vaginal discharge
- ☐ Back pain
- ☐ Swelling
- ☐ Stomach flutters

Low back pain. Your belly is beginning to protrude in ways it's never done before, and this can create a strain on your lower back. An achy soreness in your lower back that worsens during the day and resolves after sleeping through the night is typical. If you have abandoned the yoga or Pilates that you started at the beginning of pregnancy, I would recommend starting again. By keeping your core muscles strong, your body will be more in alignment, and this will keep your back pain to a minimum. Swimming is also a great exercise for back pain. Not only does it help build your core muscles, but it also provides some relief of the back pain by suspending you in the zero gravity of water.

A pregnancy support belt can also work to relieve lower back pain since it helps redistribute the belly weight. You can find these at medical supply stores or at some maternity shops. Additionally, you can try a warm bath or heating pad to relieve the pain. Yes, I did recommend you not soak in a hot tub during the first trimester; however, it is now safe to take a warm bath since baby is fully formed at this point in pregnancy. You can try acetaminophen (Tylenol), but remember to avoid anti-inflammatory medications such as ibuprofen (Advil or Motrin), as these are not safe at any time during pregnancy.

Your body is also releasing hormones that can make your joints more loose as it prepares for birth. These hormones allow your pelvis to relax, making room for the baby to pass through during delivery. Having such loose joints can, however, make them more prone to getting out of alignment. This problem can especially affect your hips. If your pain persists, consider asking for a referral to a physical therapist or chiropractor.

If back pain is associated with fever, weakness, numbness, or pain so severe that you have trouble walking, you should call your doctor. Back pain that is associated with painful urination could be a sign of a kidney infection and should be checked out immediately.

How do you know if your back pain is preterm labor? Labor pains feel like back tightness that gets more and more painful, lasting one minute and then resolving, only to return a few minutes later. If you are unsure of what you are experiencing, first try rest and acetaminophen (Tylenol). If the pain continues to get worse, notify your doctor.

Heartburn. Another common symptom at this point is heartburn. While pregnant, your body has high levels of the hormone progesterone, which brings a relaxing effect to the body. Less helpfully, it also has a relaxing effect on the valve between your stomach and esophagus. This lets the acid in your stomach pass into the sensitive lower esophagus, causing a burning sensation in your chest. Heartburn is exacerbated by the growing uterus pushing up against the stomach.

There are lots of annoying pregnancy symptoms that you just have to bear, but heartburn is one that can almost always be treated. The first step is to avoid eating for at least two hours before bed. Next, cut back on fatty and fried foods, and stay upright after eating. If these steps don't work, then take chewable calcium carbonate (such as Tums, Rolaids, or a generic equivalent). If you are still burning, famotidine (Pepcid) over-the-counter is safe to take in pregnancy. If you *still* experience symptoms, ask your doctor about prescription-strength medications.

Heartburn should be associated with eating. It should not be associated with difficulty breathing or fever. These additional symptoms should prompt a call to your doctor.

Constipation and hemorrhoids. Almost all women experience some amount of constipation during pregnancy. Constipation has been jokingly defined as having a bowel movement less often than your grandma. Medically, it's considered to be hard, painful stools, oftentimes shaped like small balls. Yes, you read that right—I have just written a full sentence about the shape of poop. But for those who suffer, it's no laughing matter. The straining from the difficult bowel movements can also lead to hemorrhoids, which are essentially swollen veins around the rectum that can also cause pain and rectal bleeding.

If you are experiencing constipation or hemorrhoids, first make sure that you are getting enough fluids and fiber. If you are getting your five servings of fruits and vegetables daily and drinking eight large glasses of water, the next step is to add a fiber supplement such as FiberCon and a stool softener. Docusate (Colace) is a safe, over-the-counter stool softener that can be taken daily. One mistake people make is stopping their stool softener once their constipation is controlled. The constipation then returns with a vengeance. If you have ongoing constipation and hemorrhoids, you should probably just stay on a stool softener daily. If you still have symptoms after making these interventions, let your doctor know because there are prescription-strength medications that can also be given.

Hemorrhoid symptoms can be safely treated with over-the-counter creams. Use moist wipes instead of toilet paper when using the bathroom to decrease discomfort. If you experience a severe or throbbing pain and swelling in your rectum, it is likely a thrombosed hemorrhoid (a small blood clot in the swollen vein). Notify your doctor or go to the emergency room, as these can usually be treated to give you instant relief.

Expectations for This Month's Visit

At this visit, your doctor will most likely begin measuring your belly, which is exactly what it sounds like. We use a soft measuring tape to measure from your pubic bone to the top of your uterus. This measurement should equal in centimeters approximately the number of weeks in your pregnancy. For example, at twenty-three weeks, your belly should measure between twenty-two and twenty-four centimeters. Your belly measurement, along with your weight gain, helps guide your doctor in knowing whether baby is growing appropriately. If your belly measurement begins to not line up with your weeks, your doctor may choose to do an additional ultrasound.

Your doctor will also listen for the baby's heartbeat. You may notice that the heartbeat is a little slower than it was in the past. Generally, baby's heartbeat will slowly decrease over time. A normal fetal heart rate is between 110 and 170. The average heart rate at the beginning of pregnancy tends to be 150 to 180, and as the baby develops neurologically, it becomes slower, averaging 120 to 150 at term. However, it is common and actually a sign of good health if the baby's heart rate varies a lot, even in the same hour.

This may be a good time to ask any specific questions you have because it is usually a brief visit.

Circumcision

If at your last visit, you found out you were having a boy, then this may be a good time to consider whether circumcision is the right choice for your son. Circumcision is considered an elective procedure (not medically necessary) by the American Academy of Pediatrics. However, the World Health Organization (WHO) has recently released a statement recommending circumcision to help prevent sexually transmitted diseases (STDs). This is a personal decision, so it is something you and your partner will need to discuss and decide what's best for your baby. It is interesting to note that the percentage of people who elect to have this done varies greatly from region to region, even within the United States.

Circumcision is usually performed the day after the baby is born, either by the OB or by the pediatrician. The current standard is to use some type of

Reasons to Consider Circumcision

- Decreased risk of urinary tract infections
- Decreased risk of STDs
- Religious considerations (for Jews or Muslims)
- Decreased risk of penile cancer (very rare)
- Social considerations (other family members have circumcision; don't want to "look different")

Reasons to Consider Not Circumcising

- Risks of the procedure (rare; include bleeding, infection, and damage to penis)
- Not considered medically necessary by American Academy of Pediatrics
- Concern over possible decrease in sexual sensitivity
- Social considerations (other members of the family not circumcised)

anesthesia for the procedure. I use a local block that involves giving a shot at the base of the penis. The procedure itself takes only a couple of minutes. Like any procedure, it involves the risk of bleeding and infection, but the risk of major complication is low.

Some groups have expressed concern as to how circumcision affects sexual function later in life. Questions have been raised as to whether removing the foreskin decreases a man's sexual sensitivity or decreases lubrication. The scientific data on the subject is minimal; in the end, the decision is up to you, and all these thoughts should be taken into consideration.[1]

VBAC

If you are considering a vaginal birth after cesarean, it is important to discuss your options with your doctor. See chapter 9 for more about VBAC and the things to consider when making this decision.

Common Questions You May Have This Month

Can I travel during pregnancy?

As long as you are not experiencing any complications in pregnancy, you can usually travel by airplane until you are thirty-five weeks along. You are more prone to blood clots forming in your legs when you are pregnant, so it is recommended that you stay well hydrated and get up and walk around every hour during long flights. This is not a problem for most pregnant women, since they usually have to pee that often anyway.

Travel by car is safe up until delivery; however, it's not recommended to go more than two hours away from your hospital after thirty-five weeks. You may go into labor and need to get there quickly. If there is a family emergency or some reason you need to travel further away, make sure you get a copy of your medical chart to have with you.

The hospital where I work is right off a major interstate, and it's not uncommon for us to have pregnant travelers pull in for delivery. I'm not sure why women would want to travel at thirty-nine weeks and deliver at an unfamiliar hospital with unfamiliar doctors, but that is a risk they take when traveling by car late in pregnancy.

Most cruise lines will not allow you to travel after twenty-five weeks. There is not really a medical reason for this, other than the fact that they don't want to deal with possible pregnancy complications in the middle of the ocean, which is understandable.

I wake up with my hands numb and tingling. Is that normal?

Yes. There is increased fluid in your tendon sheaths, which can cause a type of carpal tunnel syndrome of pregnancy. Wearing wrist splints at night can help. If the numbness persists throughout the day or you also have weakness, you may need to see a hand specialist.

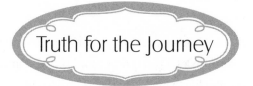

Truth for the Journey

*If you remain in me and my words remain in you, ask whatever
you wish, and it will be given you. This is to my Father's glory,
that you bear much fruit, showing yourselves to be my disciples.*

John 15:7–8

You are probably giving a sigh of relief after reading that most women are usually showing by now. It's all right to admit it. Go ahead and exhale and let that belly out! This part of your pregnancy will be fun because you are really starting to feel like a mommy-to-be. You probably feel more energized, and as you begin to feel baby moving inside your belly, you are likely becoming more and more bonded with your little one. Don't worry if these feelings do not describe you yet. Just wait, you will soon deeply connect with the fact that life is growing inside of you.

You may be concerned about how you *feel* about being pregnant at this point. Every woman responds to pregnancy differently. Some love being pregnant, flaunting their baby bellies with confidence and joy. Others are miserable, counting the days until they can get their prepregnancy body back. No matter where you fit on this spectrum of response, the reality is that you are going through many changes at a rapid pace. There is no right or wrong response to pregnancy. Try not to compare how you feel—both physically and emotionally—to other women, and try to remember that how you feel now in no way reflects how you will respond to your newborn baby. Pregnancy can take a major toll on your body and your mind. You may not be in the mood to get all gushy about baby bedding and cutesy clothes. Don't be too hard on yourself. Getting used to these changes and bonding with the idea of a little one takes time. You'll get there. In the meantime, spend as much time as you can with the Lord as you walk through this process. He will quickly come and minister to your weary body and heart.

I could never understand how most women loved being pregnant.
I felt like people judged me because I admitted I didn't like it at all. Now
that I have my son, though, I would go through all of it again in a heartbeat.
Amber, 33, mother of one

Our key Bible verse for the month comes from John 15 and talks about abiding in the vine. I can't think of a better time to wrap your mind around this concept than right now, as a life that is physically connected to you is growing at an exponential rate. What an amazing picture of how our lives (the branches) can grow and thrive as they are connected to Christ (the vine). I encourage you to read this entire chapter and meditate on the truth found there. How might it apply to your life as a mommy-to-be right now?

Our specific verses for this month say, "If you remain in me and my words remain in you, ask whatever you wish, and it will be given you. This is to my Father's glory, that you bear much fruit, showing yourselves to be my disciples" (John 15:7–8). There is so much to chew on in this passage. First, we are given a clear word that as long as we remain connected to the Lord and his Word, we can ask whatever we wish and it will be given to us. This doesn't necessarily mean that if you ask God not to gain any weight during pregnancy, it will magically happen. What it does mean is that by being connected to God and his Word, you will have a better understanding of his heart; thus, your requests will be more in line with his will. I hope this truth will be a great encouragement as you continue to ask God to protect your growing child.

What If I Hate Being Pregnant?

For those of you who would have a ton of babies if it weren't for the pregnancy part, let me address negative feelings toward pregnancy. You may feel at times as though you are the only woman in the world who doesn't like this process. That is simply not the case. I've known several women who love being a mom but hated being pregnant.

So first, I want you to understand you are not alone. Next, I want you to understand that you are not a horrible person because you don't like being pregnant. Pregnancy is a complete invasion of your body. For some women, it affects most of their functions. Don't let anyone tell you that you are wrong or will be a bad mother because you don't like being pregnant. All those women I know who hated pregnancy *love* being a mom. Be honest about your feelings, and ask God to help you enjoy it even a little bit. Our hope is that by using this book throughout your journey, you'll be able to tap into the joy and peace found in the Lord, and it will make your pregnancy much more enjoyable.

Enjoy every minute of your pregnancy, every kick, every pain, and every time you have to wake up to go to the bathroom. Thank God for what he has given you. You never know—it could be your only chance to embrace it, so take it for all that it's worth. Erica, 23, mother of one

There are so many amazing milestones this month. As Dr. Rupe mentioned, your baby is fully formed by twenty-four weeks. So even though he is only about twelve inches in length and weighs only $1\frac{1}{2}$ pounds, all of his body parts and organs are formed. Take a moment to thank God for baby's fingers and toes, for his heart and his lungs. Each of those baby parts is such a miracle. This is also the time you begin to feel baby move inside you. I will never forget the first time I felt my daughter move inside my belly. At first it felt a little odd, but after I realized what was happening, I couldn't wait for it to happen again. Those early flutters helped me feel her life in a more tangible way. And those movements reminded me to continue to bathe her growing life in prayer every day.

Since we discussed viability in this chapter, you may be experiencing a bit of anxiety about preterm labor. Be encouraged that your risk of giving birth too early is probably very low. Continue to pray and ask God to protect your baby and give you peace of mind. At this point, that is really all you can do. You may also begin to experience some discomfort due to lower back pain and other normal aspects of pregnancy. This can be very frustrating and discouraging. Make an effort to flip-flop your fear and frustration and use it to bring glory to God.

Take a look at the second of this month's verses again. "This is to my Father's glory, that you bear much fruit, *showing* yourselves to be my disciples" (italics added). In everything that we experience, we should try to figure out how it can bring God glory. When we bear fruit and *show* ourselves to be his disciples, we do just that. This pregnancy is not only a physical representation of bearing fruit; it can also be a spiritual one. Grab hold of your worries and your fears, and *show* yourself to be a confident and peace-filled expectant mom. Don't let them see you sweat. Don't let them hear you worry or complain. Use that belly of yours to *show* the world that God is good and that you believe it!

Prayer Concerns

Baby's growth and development

Mommy's comfort

Safety against preterm labor

Peace of mind

A Prayer for This Month

Dear Lord,

I want my growing belly to show of your goodness. Help me to remember your faithfulness when I feel worried or uncomfortable. As I remain connected to you, may I be filled with peace and joy and thus bring glory to you through this pregnancy. I trust you to continue to hold this baby in my womb until it is time for him to enter this world. Thank you for this precious gift of life. Amen.

Write a prayer here for your own personal journey.

Journal

Record your thoughts and your fears here. It is important to acknowledge every thought and feeling you are experiencing. The main thing is to get them out in the open, and if they do not line up with the truth or the faith that you possess, then get rid of those burdens by giving them over to your Pregnancy Companion.

Chapter Seven

Prepared to Give
Weeks 26 to 30

Key Bible Verse

Each man should give what he has decided in his heart to give, not reluctantly or under compulsion, for God loves a cheerful giver. And God is able to make all grace abound to you, so that in all things at all times, having all that you need, you will abound in every good work.

2 Corinthians 9:7–8

Baby Stats

At thirty weeks, your baby weighs in at around three pounds and is about sixteen inches long. He is almost done growing in length, so he just needs to fill out over the next couple of months. Baby's major organs are fully developed and he could, if needed, survive outside the womb, although he would need to remain in the hospital for several months. By thirty weeks, baby's toenails are fully formed.

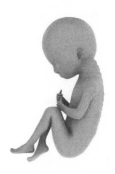

Most babies begin to develop some hair at this point. As he develops fat deposits under his skin, the skin becomes smoother and he is better able to regulate his temperature. The amount of heartburn you have does not correlate with the amount of hair on the baby, despite the views of some grandmas who would adamantly disagree with this statement.

Mommy Stats

By now, you are definitely looking pregnant. You are probably having to get used to strangers touching your tummy or making comments about when you are due. I always thought it would be fun to get a T-shirt with my due date on it. I liked a T-shirt Jessica had when she was pregnant. It said, "Hello, my name is going to be Hope," with a big arrow pointing to her growing belly. Needless to say, you are definitely "showing" by now.

At this point, you should have gained ten to fifteen pounds, and the weight should be mainly in your stomach area. If you haven't already, you might be starting to feel some heartburn.

Now would be a good time to check in to childbirth education classes. These classes are offered by most hospitals or community centers. The classes give you an overview of the birthing process and explain the epidural process (more on the epidural later). Even if you are having a cesarean section, I recommend childbirth classes because they help familiarize you with the whole hospital process. If you desire natural childbirth, then you should consider more in-depth Lamaze or Bradley method classes. The hospital classes will only give you an overview; they are not intended specifically to prepare you for natural childbirth.

Deciding on your method of pain control is an important thing to begin considering. I have a lot of patients who say, "I'll try going natural, but I want to leave the door open for an epidural." I've never seen any of them go natural! Labor is called *labor* for a reason. It is very intense. If you decide that having a natural childbirth is important to you, then you need to be prepared and have an excellent support system with you. We'll address your options further in Chapter Eight.

Symptom Checker

- ☐ Constipation or hemorrhoids
- ☐ Heartburn
- ☐ Backaches
- ☐ Enlarged breasts
- ☐ Swelling
- ☐ Leg cramps
- ☐ Bleeding gums
- ☐ Shortness of breath
- ☐ Sleeplessness
- ☐ Clumsiness
- ☐ Fetal movement
- ☐ Occasional contractions

You should continue to exercise at this point in the pregnancy. You should still have a fair amount of energy. You may not feel very energetic, but you have more energy now than you'll have in another few months. So, this is a good time for any major projects like getting the nursery ready or visiting out-of-state relatives.

Movement, movement, movement. Can that baby ever move! At this point in the pregnancy, the baby is very active. Your family and friends can probably feel the movements through your belly. The movement is a sign that the baby is happy and healthy inside you. When the baby has the hiccups, it means he's especially healthy. Hiccups are a great sign that the baby's nervous system is developing normally.

Starting at twenty-seven weeks, you should begin counting movements (kick counts). A *movement* is a definite kick or turn of the baby. Twice a day, count how many times the baby moves in an hour. Baby needs to move at least six times an hour. You don't need to count every hour of the day, and you can stop counting when you get to six. If you don't count six movements in an hour, then eat

Kick Count Chart

Don't forget to count 2 times per day. Your baby should move at least 6 times per hour.										
Date	Time	1	2	3	4	5	6	7	8	9	10
4/10	1-2pm	x	x	x	x	x	x	x	x		

something sweet and lie on your side and recount. If you still don't count six, you should call your doctor immediately. If there is something wrong with the baby, the first detectable symptom is a decrease in movement.

I had a patient come to an appointment after I'd told her about kick counts with a detailed spreadsheet including all her baby's movements graphed over the month. One day, she counted 150 movements in an hour. The next day, it was 200. I reassured her that she could stop counting at six, and she didn't need to bring them in. She can save her graphing for the pediatrician!

Expectations for This Month's Visit

The next visit will most likely include your diabetes screen. Before your diabetes test, there is no need to fast or change your diet. You will be given a sugary drink, and your blood will be drawn an hour after you drink it. If you do not pass this test, you will have to take a three-hour confirmatory test. The confirmation test requires an overnight fast.

In pregnancy, the placenta secretes several different hormones. One is called *insulin-like growth factor*, and as you get further along, the placenta gets bigger and secretes more of this hormone. The hormone causes your body to need more insulin to process its carbohydrates, sometimes to the point that you become diabetic. This type of diabetes can usually be controlled with diet and also usually resolves after delivery, when you get rid of the placenta. Exercise is beneficial to help prevent gestational diabetes because it helps your body process insulin more efficiently. Sometimes, despite following the diet and exercise, you will still not be able to keep your sugars in the normal range. This is not your fault; rather, it is the fault of the extra hormones being secreted by the placenta and the result of how they interact with your body.

The good thing about gestational diabetes is that it is not necessarily permanent. It will usually resolve within days of birth. At your six-week postpartum checkup, however, you will need another glucose test to confirm that it has resolved. Those who have had gestational diabetes are at higher risk to develop type 2 diabetes later in life, so it is important to continue to watch your diet and be tested yearly for diabetes.

If your blood type is Rh-negative, you may also be getting your RhoGAM shot at this visit. About fifteen percent of Caucasians have an Rh-negative blood type (it's uncommon in other ethnicities). If the father of the baby is Rh-positive, then the baby could have a positive blood type. When such a baby is born, his blood can enter the mother's bloodstream and act almost like a virus, causing the mother to form an immunity against the Rh-positive blood. This situation doesn't affect the current pregnancy, but it may affect future pregnancies. The body's immune system can begin to attack the baby's blood, causing major complications. The RhoGAM shot acts to bind any Rh-positive blood that enters the mom's bloodstream and prevent the reaction from happening. It's usually given at twenty-eight weeks, but it should be given earlier if there is any bleeding or trauma during your pregnancy.

If you have this blood type, your doctor will talk to you early in pregnancy about the importance of this shot, but remember to let her know earlier if you have any bleeding. Let me clarify that you should call your doctor if you are experiencing *vaginal* bleeding. I recently received an after-hours call from a patient who had cut her finger and was bleeding. She was concerned that she needed her RhoGAM shot. I reassured her that only placental or vaginal bleeding is an issue.

Preparing to Breastfeed

Now is the time to think about preparing for breastfeeding. The list of the benefits of breastfeeding could fill this entire page. It has been shown to reduce the risk of infection in infancy, as well as the risk of chronic disease later in the child's life. For the mother, it improves bonding with the child and leads to maternal weight loss.

If breastfeeding is so great, why do nearly seventy percent of women stop before the baby is six months old? For something so natural, it's not always easy. For lots of women, the baby latches on without difficulty, feeds, grows, and flourishes. For others, it is a painful, challenging, and stressful process. The current recommendation of the American Academy of Pediatrics is to breastfeed for at least a year. This may not be possible in all situations, but it can at least be a goal.

For some of you, breastfeeding is not going to work out, and bottle-feeding will be the right choice. That is OK. Now is the time to consider whether breastfeeding may be a good choice for you and your family.

Breastfeeding		Bottle-Feeding	
Pros	**Cons**	**Pros**	**Cons**
• Improved immune response in baby • Reduced risk of SIDS • Reduced obesity • It's free • Maternal weight loss after delivery • Improved bonding	• Painful at first • Can be difficult to return to work and pump • Mastitis • Unable to switch off feeding with partner	• Easy • Can trade off responsibilities at night (better sleep for mom) • Know exactly how much baby is getting with each feeding • Makes returning to work easier	• Expensive • Constant bottle washing • Doesn't give the immunity boost that breastfeeding does

Once you have decided on your feeding method, planning ahead is helpful. If you have specific concerns, then meeting with a lactation consultant before delivery can be helpful.[1] Review the following chart, and if you fall under the category of needing additional help breastfeeding, you definitely will want to meet with a lactation consultant before delivery.

Prevents Breastfeeding	Affects Ability to Breastfeed (you may need additional help)	Does Not Affect Ability to Breastfeed
• HIV positive • Tuberculosis • Active chicken pox or shingles on breast • Cytomegalovirus (CMV) • Hepatitis • Illicit drug use	• Breast reduction • Lumpectomy • Treatment for breast cancer • Tubular shaped breasts • Significantly asymmetric breasts • PCOS • Inverted nipples	• Breast augmentation • Pierced nipples • Smoking • Very small or very large breasts

Common Questions You May Have This Month

Do I need to take a prenatal class?

Did you drive a car before someone taught you how? Maybe I'm crazy, but I wouldn't want to go through the shock of having a baby without someone walking me through it first! Nobody will hold a gun to your head and make you take a prenatal class, but we recommend that you do. The classes cover everything from nutrition to labor to pain management to taking care of a newborn. Especially if you've never done this before, prenatal classes will explain some of the most valuable information you will have access to during your pregnancy.

Check with your hospital to see if and when they offer the class. It is helpful to take a class at the hospital because it will likely include information about labor and delivery at that facility. However, it is likely there are many other classes offered in your city. Check out www.icea.org for a list of accredited childbirth educators in your area.

I've noticed a dark line down my belly. Is that normal?
Yes. Women often get increased pigmentation (darkening of skin) in several areas of their body, including their vulva, their underarms, and down the middle of their belly. This darkening is more pronounced in women who are of darker skin tone. It normally lightens after delivery.

How do I know if I am experiencing preterm labor?
As you near the end of your pregnancy, you will likely experience many odd cramps and twinges. I'm sure every woman has thought at some point toward the end that she was having preterm labor. Because every body and every pregnancy is so different, it is hard to say how you will know if you are experiencing signs of preterm labor (see page 212 for more on signs of preterm labor). If you are experiencing tightening in your abdomen that comes and goes, rest and increase your fluid intake. If the tightening doesn't go away, then call your doctor.

The Doctor's POV: Gestational Diabetes

I find that most patients really dread their diabetes test. I'm not sure why. Maybe it's the glucola drink. The drinks we have today are not too bad, and the test usually requires only one blood draw. Now, *failing* the diabetes test *is* probably something to dread. The confirmatory test requires fasting, drinking a stronger drink, and four blood draws. Yeah . . . much less fun.

Gestational diabetes is one area of pregnancy where I feel I can really make a difference. If left untreated, gestational diabetes can cause significant complications, such as babies that are so big that they get stuck in the birth canal. It can even lead to stillbirth. The good news is that by diagnosing and treating gestational diabetes, which usually involves simple dietary changes, these babies can have a perfectly normal delivery. Treating gestational diabetes can make a huge difference in the health of your baby, so although the test is an inconvenience, it's the first of many that you'll experience in an effort to take care of your baby.

When I was pregnant, I craved orange soda, so I actually thought the glucola drink tasted good. Likewise, since I did crave so much soda, I was a little worried I would fail the test. But thankfully, I passed.

The Patient's POV: Gestational Diabetes

Because I have a condition called polycystic ovary syndrome (PCOS), Dr. Rupe always knew I would be at high risk for gestational diabetes. I was tested very early in my pregnancy (around twelve weeks). Typically, expectant mothers are not tested until somewhere around weeks twenty-four to twenty-eight. Although I prayed and prayed that I would not have gestational diabetes, one afternoon I received the dreaded call that I did have it. I hung up the phone and cried, feeling so sorry for myself. I immediately called my girlfriend, and I will never forget what she said. "Jess, I think this is going to be a gift from God." In the moment, those words did make me feel better, even though I had no idea how true they would become.

The news came right before Christmas, so you can imagine my disappointment that there would be no holiday sweets for me. Dr. Rupe sent me to a nutritionist, and I was put on a strict low-carb diet. I had to prick my finger four times a day, eat at very specific times, and report every single thing I put into my mouth to Dr. Rupe at the end of each week. If my blood sugar rose, it could affect the baby, and Dr. Rupe needed to know it.

Six months later, I gave birth to a very healthy baby. Although I went into my pregnancy a bit overweight, I was healthier after giving birth than I was before I had gotten pregnant. Most women don't get the chance to say that. While it's true that gestational diabetes can be a pain in the you-know-what, God can use it—as he does most things—to your benefit. If you happen to be one of the one percent of pregnant women who are diagnosed with gestational diabetes, don't let it get you down. Consider it an opportunity to take extra care of your body during your pregnancy.

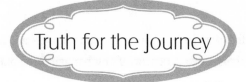
Truth for the Journey

Each man should give what he has decided in his heart to give, not reluctantly or under compulsion, for God loves a cheerful giver. And God is able to make all grace abound to you, so that in all things at all times, having all that you need, you will abound in every good work.
2 Corinthians 9:7–8

Preparing for Baby

By now you may have the nursery all ready to welcome your little one. You may have registered at your favorite baby store for all that stuff they say you need but you're not sure you need. You might be a little exhausted and overwhelmed by everything that comes with welcoming a new life into your home. The best advice I can give you is—don't panic! Babies were born long before bouncy seats and swings, fancy strollers and play yards. There's little your baby really needs beyond food, shelter, clothing and, of course, love. But every expectant mom goes through these necessary preparations with great joy and trepidation. The important thing is to keep your head on straight and remember that you need to keep first things first.

Perhaps the most important point of preparation during these forty weeks is that you become spiritually ready to parent this child. Don't get me wrong: no one expects you to be perfectly prepared for the major life change that lies ahead. However, there are steps you can take to prepare yourself for the most important role of your life. I don't know if I ever felt completely ready to parent, no matter how much time we spent reflecting on the road ahead. Of course, the grace of God was with me, and the Lord quickly showed me ways to be a good parent. He'll do the same for you, and we've included a few steps you can take early on to point you in the right direction.

Spend time in the Word. Nothing, nothing, nothing will prepare you more for any major life change than the Word of God. He's covered it all in the Bible! From practical parenting advice to simple words of encouragement to prime parental examples, it's all in there! I encourage you to find time daily to dig in to the Word and seek out its parenting stories and instruction. Here are a few examples to get you started:

- 2 Corinthians 9:7–8 (our key verse for this month)
- 2 Corinthians 12:9 (reminding us that his grace is sufficient)
- Colossians 3:12–17 (great instruction for living a life of love and peace)
- James 1:5–8 (ask him for wisdom and he will give it to you)

Lean into other moms. One of the greatest resources you have around you is other moms. They may all do things a bit differently and have somewhat different approaches to parenting, but I'd venture to guess that if you pay close attention, you'll learn something great from each and every one of them. The important thing is to take what you hear or observe and then ask God for discernment as you determine what is right for your family. There are only a few nonnegotiable things when it comes to parenting—those addressed in the Bible, such as love, discipline, and training your child according to God's Word. Once those things are established, everything else is really about preference and what works best for you.

When I was in my third trimester, I made an appointment to spend the day with one of my best friends who was a mother of two children under four years old. I observed, asked questions, and walked away with a lot to chew on regarding my own family. This is just one example of the hours I spent listening, observing, and asking questions of my mothering girlfriends. I received a wealth of knowledge and insight I could never have found in a book. This practice didn't end when my baby arrived. Actually, it got more intense. I like to call the first few months of parenting *trial by fire*. I wanted as many friends in the fire with me as possible. I regularly called or e-mailed my girlfriends to ask them questions about feeding, scheduling, toys, and gear. There are no better examples than those who have gone before. Take advantage of the wealth of knowledge in your sphere. If nothing else, talking to other moms will help you realize you are not crazy as you navigate the uncharted waters of motherhood.

Talk it out. With all of the emotional and physical adjustments that come with being a new parent, perhaps the most dangerous reaction is to keep it all inside. God gave you a partner in your spouse or perhaps a family member or friend with whom you are walking through your pregnancy. He desires for you to join together in caring for this child. Just because you are the mom, it doesn't mean it's all up to you. The most important thing for your family is unity between you and your support system. When baby is up all night crying, you must be united. When baby gets sick for the first time, even if you don't know what to do, you must be united. The only way this unity can come is through lots of prayer and lots of talking!

I know that many men do not naturally open up, especially when they are experiencing something new and possibly scary. If this is the case in your situation, I encourage you to gently nudge your spouse to a place of openness. Begin asking questions. Ask him to share what he is feeling. If that seems like a long shot, ask something more specific, such as:

- Who do you think our little one will look like?
- Are you afraid of changing baby's diaper or dressing him?
- What is the one thing you look forward to in the coming year?
- What do you think you'll enjoy about being a daddy? What scares you?

These questions, if nothing else, will get him talking. Once he begins discussing his thoughts and feelings, you'll likely be able to go deeper. Simply take what you know of your husband and his personality and start slowly, moving in the direction of complete openness when it comes to your family.

Journal your thoughts, both joys and fears. Before I got pregnant, I had fantasy-like visions of preparing a daily journal for my unborn child. I just knew I would record my innermost thoughts and dreams for my baby in a beautiful little book that I would present to her when she was old enough to appreciate it. Needless to say, I have no book to present. I think the whole idealistic view of journaling made it that much more intimidating to me, so I didn't follow through completely. I did write down occasional thoughts and fears, and I also kept a weekly blog for those friends and family following our journey.

My point is . . . don't put too much pressure on yourself to do it like they do it in the movies. I have news for you: it's a lot easier when it's written in the script, and the script is written by a professional screenwriter. Give yourself a break. It doesn't have to be perfect. It has to be *you*. Do whatever you feel the grace to do during your season of pregnancy. Whatever it is, it will be special to you and to your child if you choose to share it with him someday.

More important than the legacy of journaling during your pregnancy is the therapy of journaling. Make it more about getting your thoughts out of your head and on paper. If you are like me, you'll have millions of thoughts popping in and out of your head while you are pregnant. For some of us, this isn't too far off from normal. But add in those pregnancy hormones, and you'll find your mind wandering all over the place. Take some time to record those thoughts— both joys and fears—and in doing so, submit them to the Father. He'll quickly come and bathe them in his perfect peace. Journaling is about taking personal time to deal with everything that is going through your head. Do yourself a favor and get it out!

> Enjoy every kick no matter how uncomfortable they may be. You will never be pregnant with this baby again. Melinda, 35, mother of two

Treasure this time. You will never hold your child this close ever again. I know you've already sensed the amazing gift it is to be able to carry a child within your womb. Just remember that this time will pass by quickly, and although you'll likely be the closest human being to your little one, you will never again hold him like this, as a new life growing inside of you—receiving everything he needs directly from you. Treasure this time. You are part of an amazing miracle.

In the Gospel of Luke, we read the story of the birth of Jesus and see how Mary reacted in the midst of such a miraculous event. Luke 2:19 says, "But Mary treasured up all these things and pondered them in her heart."

Learn from Mary's response. Treasure this time and really think about the miracle you are holding inside of you. If God is able to perform this great miracle of life, he is more than able to give you all the grace and strength you need to be a parent.

Stewardship and Budgeting

Web sites and checklists. Customer reviews and safety recalls. There is so much information out there these days about which new, super baby gadgets you just have to have and those you should just stay away from. There are books and Web sites devoted to helping you find the best deals. I know, because I used them all! My husband and I are suckers for a deal, and we spent hours searching for the best price on everything from strollers to chandeliers. But while I am a proponent for bargain shopping, I encourage you to keep things in perspective and, again, keep first things first.

Each of us will welcome a child into our homes during different seasons of our lives. Some will be just starting out in marriage. Some will be more established, having waited a bit longer to begin a family. And some may be single parents, facing the responsibility of the baby alone. Whatever your story, stewardship must be the goal.

I love the teaching of Jesus in Luke 12:22–34. He begins this teaching (often titled "Do Not Worry") with the verse, "Therefore I tell you, do not worry about your life, what you will eat; or about your body, what you will wear." He is clearly challenging his followers to take their focus off material things. He goes on to give examples of how the heavenly Father meets the needs of every living creature. He then states boldly, "But seek his kingdom, and these things will be given to you as well." Another promise of provision. Lastly, he implores us to sell our possessions and give to the poor, making only for ourselves treasures in heaven. This teaching ends with one of Jesus' most quoted scriptures, "For where your treasure is, there your heart will be also."

You don't need every fancy contraption sold on the market to have a happy baby. A diaper, a blanket, and some milk will do just fine. Annrose, 35, mother of two

There is so much in this teaching to digest, but I believe so much of the message is about stewardship. Stewardship in its most raw form is simply about balance. Do not worry. Trust in God. Put others before yourself. Seek him first and he will provide. As you trust God for provision and for wisdom in how to prepare physically for your child, seek him first and you will achieve the balance of good stewardship.

What should stewardship look like in your home? Well, that greatly depends on the season of life you are in. But even if your household has plenty of money coming in, you don't necessarily need to spend a lot on baby. And similarly, even if your household is on a tighter budget, you don't need to settle for less.

My husband and I welcomed our first child almost six years into our marriage. We had a little extra money at the time because I was working, so we did invest in things like furniture, but that didn't stop me from searching out every deal I could find. I was going to let myself spend a little more on bedding because I couldn't find anything I liked. I decided on a certain designer that had baby bedding in her collection. It was a bit on the pricey side, but I told myself it would be one of the few things we splurged on. Less than twenty-four hours after I chose the bedding I wanted, I found it online at fifty percent off! You see, stewardship is not about settling for less. It's about wisdom and savvy when it comes to spending.

You might be wondering why I am addressing this issue in a pregnancy book. You probably figure most people spend what they can spend, and that's that. I think establishing a foundation of stewardship in the home is more than just living within a budget and is an important first step. If you haven't taken this step already, why not start with baby's arrival? Having a baby is likely one of the most expensive things you've had to deal with in your life. Now is the time to establish your family's financial values. You will be carrying an extra financial responsibility for the next eighteen or more years. You'd better learn to deal with it in a Godly manner!

Baby Needs

Open any pregnancy book or magazine, and you'll likely find a list of baby items to consider. It can be very overwhelming to peruse that list. Strollers, bottles, car seats. You might be wondering: What exactly does baby need? How many of those should I get? And what exactly is a Boppy, anyway? Do I really need one?

For the sake of simplicity and organization, I'd like to break down these common lists into three categories. The "Must" Haves. The "Would Be Nice" to Haves. And the "Everyone in Hollywood" Haves. You'll find a corresponding budget worksheet in the Appendix at the end of this book. I encourage you to spend time with these lists, considering them in regard to your own preferences and lifestyle. This is certainly a very exciting time in your life, and you deserve to enjoy the fun of new baby gear. Just to keep it in perspective . . . try this . . . the other day it dawned on me that all the stuff I spent hours mulling over my daughter used for less than a year! It's all packed up in a closet somewhere. So much of it didn't even matter!

What does baby really need? Not much, really! Most of it is up to your personal preferences and the systems you create in your home to make life with baby as easy as possible for you.

Level One Needs
The "Must" Haves

Furniture/Nursery
Crib, Crib mattress, Crib bumper, Changing table or dresser (combine these two to save money), Rocker or chair

Gear
Car seat, Stroller, Diaper bag, Toys

Feeding
Breast pump, Bottles, OR, Bottles, Formula, Pacifiers

Diapering
Diapers (cloth or disposable), Wipes, Diaper covers (if using cloth), Changing pad and cover, Garbage pail, Diaper rash cream, Thermometer

Bathing

Tub (or something to bathe baby on. Bath sponges are great and inexpensive!), Towels, Washcloths, Baby shampoo or body wash, Grooming kit

Linens

Crib sheets, Blankets, Bibs, Burp cloths, Mattress protector

Clothing

Onesies (long- and short-sleeved), T-shirts, Pants, Pajamas, Sweater Socks or booties, Hat, Jacket, Hangers

Level Two Needs
The "Would Be Nice" to Haves

In addition to the items listed in level one, it would be nice to have these items if your budget allows.

Furniture/Nursery

Crib bedding set, Nursery décor, Mobile, Hamper

Gear

Bouncy seat, Activity gym, Play yard, Baby monitor, Swing, Sling or carrier

Feeding

Storage bags, Nursing bra, Nipple cream, Nursing or support pillow, Nursing cover, OR, Formula dispenser, Bottle brush, Drying rack , Dishwasher basket

Diapering

Diaper pail and stacker, Extra changing pad covers

Bathing

Rubber ducky

Linens

Extra crib sheets, Sheet savers, Play yard sheets, Blankets of varying weights

Clothing

Special outfit for leaving the hospital, Going out outfit

Level Three "Needs"
The "Everyone in Hollywood" Haves

And if there isn't enough already, some people actually get these things for baby.

Gear
Stroller system, Jogging stroller, Rain cover for stroller, Sun shades for car, Crib and/or car mirror, Stroller/car seat toys, Digital camera, Video camera

Feeding
Electric breast pump, OR, Sterilizer, Bottle warmer

Diapering
Wipe warmer

Bathing
Bath thermometer

Linens
Ultimate crib sheet (I'll explain more later)

Clothing
Expensive boutique outfits

Getting a Good Deal
Depending on where you live, you may have a choice of baby superstores in your area. It is important to scope out your options early to find the one with the best deals. Make sure you ask the sales associates about special discounts and programs for joining their mailing list or baby registry. You'll be surprised and annoyed by how much baby spam you get in the mail after you sign up for your first Web site or program. But don't knock it! You may be overwhelmed by all those coupons flooding your mailbox, but you will likely use them.

When looking for a deal, the important thing to remember is don't take anything at face value. Don't ever pay full price for anything. The World Wide Web is your door into the world of bargain hunting. You can also use a cell phone app such as ShopSavvy or RedLaser to scan barcodes right in the store and search immediately online for a better price. You should never have to pay top dollar for anything. It might take a tad bit more time to do the research, but your wallet will thank you.

Baby Bargains. My friend Kristy was a great resource when I was pregnant. She turned me on to all kinds of books and Web sites and places to get a deal. One of the most incredible resources she gave me was a book called *Baby Bargains* by Denise Fields and Alan Fields. Packed with information and very simply organized, *Baby Bargains* covers every major purchase (and even some minor ones) you will make for baby with product reviews, costs, and tips on how to save money. Before I read this book, I was dead set on the crib I wanted. Once I got my hands on this tool, I quickly looked it up to see what they had to say. Sadly, my crib had received an F rating because the company had seen hundreds of recalls in the past few years. I did not purchase this crib. But the book helped me find the one I did purchase, giving me lots of tips that led me to my decision. There are several books on the market like this one, so shop around for the one that best meets your needs. The main takeaway here is to do your research!

Consignment sales. I have just recently entered the crazy world of "mommy consignment sale-ing." Let me just tell you, this world is not for the faint of heart. Oh no. You will be pushed, shoved, and beaten in an effort to get to that $20 Bumbo chair, but you will have saved $40, so it will be worth it! The opportunities to save are endless in the consignment sale world if you are willing to deal with countless other moms looking for the same deals you are. You will likely get up at the crack of dawn, and you will definitely stand in line, but you could potentially walk away with everything you need for baby for a fraction of the retail cost, not to mention making money yourself when you are ready to sell your own baby items.

Consignment sales are very hit or miss. You may attend one and completely score, finding everything on your wish list. Or you might attend one and come up with nothing. Look for various sales in your area and check them out. I'm sure you'll find some are better than others, and you'll quickly learn which sales to frequent. Once you have baby and later have plenty of his clothes and gear to sell, you should be able to receive special offers and access as a consignor yourself. Check out www.kidsconsignmentsales.com for a list of sales all across the U.S.

Craigslist. If you have craigslist in your area and have not yet used it, or if you are not sure whether you have a local craigslist, put down this book, go online, and visit www.craigslist.org.

The first thing my husband and I bought for our baby was a rocker and ottoman for the nursery. I knew I wanted a full-on upholstered chair and ottoman, but they ranged from $700 to over $1000 for the set at most stores. I happened to look on craigslist one day, just to see if people sold this kind of thing. I found a listing for a chair and ottoman in perfect condition. It happened to be in the next town over (so not much of a drive) and was selling for $300 for the set! First come, first served on these sites, so I immediately e-mailed and made an appointment to pick it up that night. We saved over $400!

The downside to craigslist is that you have to be ready to buy, and you'll likely have to drive to the seller's location to take a look at the product. Don't feel pressured to purchase it, however, if it is not up to par or you just don't like it. If the chair had been covered in stains or torn, we would have passed. Because it was in perfect condition, we decided to buy it. But we had to take it on the spot or risk losing it to another buyer.

You can find all kinds of things on craigslist, from strollers to cribs to complete baby wardrobes. My friend once listed free diapers because her daughter had grown out of them, and they were just sitting in her closet. She wanted to bless someone, and I'd venture to guess the single mom who claimed them became a huge craigslist shopper after that, if she wasn't already.

Coupons, coupons, coupons. As soon as you found out you were pregnant, I'm pretty sure you signed up for several e-mail lists that promise you weekly progress reports and pregnancy tips. I know I did! Babycenter.com. Pregnancyweekly. com. There are several sites out there that provide great, free information for you and your growing baby. Go ahead and sign up because the information is always timely and very useful. However, I will warn you that the minute you type in your personal information, you will begin receiving huge amounts of pregnancy propaganda in the mail. Right now, this may seem like an unwelcome nuisance, but don't grab the recycle bin too quickly. Much of this information will be very helpful, not to mention the coupons!

For personal reasons (some beyond my control) my baby girl was formula fed. I'm not sure if you've done the research yet, but formula is pretty expensive. Although we had room in the budget and prepared for this expense, I cannot tell you how excited we were every time we received a package from Enfamil with several $5-off coupons. Five dollars off! That's amazing. We're not talking pennies here, people. We are talking a cup of Starbucks coffee or a cute pair of earrings at Target off each can of formula we purchased. And the most amazing thing is, the coupons kept coming. Thank you, Enfamil!

There are many companies that have programs like this. Pampers, Huggies, Gerber, Similac. Sign up with all of them! You will get mail from each of the companies you sign up with, but the information they send is actually very helpful, and the coupons make it all worth it. Oh, and I almost forgot to mention—not only do these companies send you coupons, but some of them send samples as well! Woo hoo!

The power of Google. My husband and I are googlin' fools! We google everything! We never make a purchase (in store or online) without googling the product first to see who has the best price. Simply make it a new habit to assume you can find a better price if you look online. You may not always find a better price, but it's best to believe you will and do the legwork necessary to save. Even a few dollars adds up in the end.

Amazon.com. I'm pretty sure if you graphed my spending for the past two to three years, the majority of it has been on Amazon.com. Much like our Google discipline, we also check Amazon.com before making a purchase. Chances are they have it cheaper (even if just a few dollars less) and likely offer free shipping and no tax on the item. I also discovered a program on Amazon called Subscribe & Save. I now have my diapers delivered right to my door once a month. I pay a few dollars less than in the store with free shipping and no tax! You just can't beat that. Not only am I saving money, but I am also saving time and the stress of realizing we are about to be out of diapers. Amazon offers a program called Amazon

Mom as well. It's free to sign up, and they offer an even bigger discount on diapers (thirty percent off) to moms who join this program and Subscribe & Save.

Retailmenot.com. This fabulous Web site is one of many that offers the opportunity to search for online coupon codes. If you didn't know this already, one of the first rules of online shopping is to never purchase anything online without searching for a coupon code first. Retailmenot.com makes it easy to do so. There are many coupons floating out there on the Internet. Make sure you look for them before buying anything.

Baby registries. Hopefully, one of your family members or friends is going to throw a shower to help you prepare for your little one. And when there is a shower, there is a baby registry (or registries)! Registering for our baby was one of the most fun things I've ever done. Picking out things that other people will buy us— who doesn't love that? As mentioned, my hubby and I love to research products, so a lot of thought went into everything we scanned with that fun little gun. I looked forward to the day of my shower, anticipating all the wonderful gear I'd get to lug home. My shower was absolutely beautiful, and I was completely overwhelmed by the blessing of it all, but inevitably many of the women couldn't help but buy me cute baby girl clothes, and so much of that wonderful gear was left at the store. But perhaps the coolest thing about registering is that most stores offer an incentive for you to come back and purchase anything you did not receive for ten percent or fifteen percent off the regular price. This is another great way to save as you invest in everything you will need for baby. Pay close attention to the registry policy at the stores you choose. Make sure they offer this incentive as, nowadays, most stores do!

As I was asking God to show me what truth he would have me share with you this month, I was led back to the key Bible verse. This passage has encouraged me through the years when I was in the midst of a situation I didn't think I could handle. Although the verse refers to financial giving, I believe the heart behind it applies to anything we are giving our life to. I'll repeat it again here. Hey, at this rate, you'll have it memorized by the time this chapter is through!

"Each man should give what he has decided in his heart to give, not reluctantly or under compulsion, for God loves a cheerful giver. And God is able to make all grace abound to you, so that in all things at all times, having all that you need, you will abound in every good work" (2 Cor. 9:7–8).

You will abound, my friend, as you prepare to parent, because God is able. Go forth diligently and confidently, knowing his grace is sufficient for you.

Prayer Concerns

Baby's growth and development
Mommy's health
Being spiritually ready for baby
Our baby budget

A Prayer for This Month

Dear Lord,

There are so many things to get ready for. Being a good parent, a good steward. It's all a bit overwhelming. Help me, Lord, to keep my eyes fixed on you as I walk this road. Give me wisdom and discernment to make the right choices. I trust that you will provide everything we need for baby. I thank you in advance for that abundant provision. Please prepare my heart to lead this child well. I know I have everything I need in your Word and through you, my Companion. Thank you, heavenly Father, for the great example I have in you and your Son. Amen.

Write a prayer here for your own personal journey.

_____

_____

_____

_____

_____

Journal

Record your thoughts and your fears here. It is important to acknowledge every thought and feeling you are experiencing. The main thing is to get them out in the open, and if they do not line up with the truth or the faith that you possess, then get rid of those burdens by giving them over to your Pregnancy Companion.

_____

_____

_____

_____

_____

Chapter Eight

Deliver Me!
Weeks 31 to 35

Key Bible Verse

But he said to me, 'My grace is sufficient for you, for my power is made perfect in weakness.' Therefore I will boast all the more gladly about my weaknesses, so that Christ's power may rest on me.

2 Corinthians 12:9

Baby Stats

Your baby is beginning to fill out. He is around 5¾ pounds and eighteen inches long by thirty-five weeks. Babies generally gain half a pound a week from thirty-two to thirty-eight weeks, and then the weight gain begins to slow down. He is developing a layer of fat under the skin, which will aid in maintaining his temperature after he is born. He is beginning to grow less in length and instead grow more in weight. His fingernails are growing and hardening. His skin is covered with a thick layer of a creamy substance called vernix. This provides protection from being in the watery environment of your amniotic sac all the time.

Baby's movements are pronounced, but they will begin to change somewhat as he grows and starts to run out of room in there. Don't forget to continue your movement counts! By thirty-five weeks, he has picked a position, either head first (ninety-seven percent of the time) or butt first (three percent of the time). Baby's position at thirty-five weeks is usually his position at term. This is one of the things your doctor will check at your thirty-five-week visit. Breech (butt first) babies cannot be safely born vaginally. So if your baby is breech, your doctor will discuss the options of cesarean section and external version (where the doctor physically flips the baby by pushing through your abdomen).

Mommy Stats

Welcome to the home stretch! I mean this literally . . . as you will most likely have a few stretch marks by this time. I always bragged that I didn't have any stretch marks, only to discover after I delivered that I was just so big I couldn't see them! There is no magic potion to prevent stretch marks. Trying to stay a healthy weight and using a moisturizing lotion that contains shea butter can be helpful. If you do develop stretch marks, you can blame your mom, because they are mostly genetic. However, she in turn can blame *you* for hers.

At this point in pregnancy, there is no hiding the belly, so you might as well try to enjoy it. When else in your life can you completely exhale and not worry about your belly fat? You may notice a return of fatigue. This may be due to difficulty sleeping or the fact that you are carrying around an extra twenty-five pounds. It's normal to begin to feel more tired at this point, so try to rest as much as possible.

You may also find that your bladder is behaving in strange ways. Depending on the position of the baby, there may be a tiny baby part pushing on or kicking your bladder. This will cause you to have to go more often, or cause you to leak some urine if you cough or sneeze. These symptoms almost always resolve after delivery. You may want to go ahead and check out the Kegel exercises. These exercises will help keep your pelvic floor muscles strong. As long as there is a baby sitting on your bladder, however, you will continue to have some bladder issues.

Kegel Exercises

Kegel exercises help strengthen the muscles that control your bowel and bladder functions. You don't want to tighten your abdominal muscles or thigh muscles. To make sure you are using the right muscles, it is best initially to do these exercises while you are peeing. Begin to pee, then contract your muscles to make the stream stop. Hold the muscles tight for ten seconds, then release. Repeat ten times. Once you have learned the correct muscles to use, you can do Kegels anywhere. Doing three sets of ten is a good start.

Symptom Checker

- ☐ Constipation or hemorrhoids
- ☐ Heartburn
- ☐ Backaches
- ☐ Enlarged breasts
- ☐ Swelling
- ☐ Leg cramps
- ☐ Returned frequent urination
- ☐ Colostrum
- ☐ Bleeding gums
- ☐ Sleeplessness
- ☐ Clumsiness
- ☐ Fetal movement
- ☐ Occasional contractions

Colostrum. Your breasts have most likely increased by at least a cup size at this point. It is normal for breasts to be asymmetric, so don't be worried if they look a bit off. You may also be experiencing some leakage from your breasts. This fluid is called colostrum, the precursor to your breast milk. It is usually white or clear and will come from multiple ducts. If you notice bloody discharge or discharge that comes from a single duct, you should be examined by your doctor.

Breast soreness. Some women may also have nipple soreness. You can purchase lanolin cream to use for sore nipples during breastfeeding. This also works well for nipple soreness during pregnancy. Make sure you have a well-fitting bra. You may need new bras at several points during pregnancy, so it's a good idea to go to a bra shop (or maternity shop) every three months to get measured. Properly fitting bras will reduce back pain and chafing. Hold on to the bras you outgrow. You may fit back into them after delivery, on your way back down to your prepregnancy weight.

Swelling. Up to seventy percent of pregnant women experience swelling during their pregnancy, the majority toward the final weeks. Swelling is commonly found in your hands and feet. As long as your blood pressure is normal and the swelling is symmetric, this is considered a routine symptom. If the swelling is significantly worse on one side, or if the swelling doesn't resolve with rest, then contact your physician, as this could be a sign of a blood clot in your leg. The best way to alleviate swelling—or at least the discomfort you feel from it—is to rest and drink lots of water.

Braxton Hicks contractions. You will likely begin to have some contractions at this point in pregnancy. These "practice contractions" are referred to as *Braxton Hicks contractions*. They were named after the English doctor who first discovered them in 1872. My bet is a lot of women "discovered" them way before that. Some will feel like a muscle tightening; others may actually make you stop what you're doing and take a deep breath. Having one or two non-painful contractions in an hour is normal. If you notice more than a couple in an hour, then drink some extra water and try to rest. The same hormone that tells your body that you are dehydrated can tell your uterus to contract. If the contractions become more regular despite rest and fluids, then call your doctor.

Expectations for This Month's Visit

At thirty weeks, you usually start visiting your doctor every two weeks. At thirty-five weeks, you will begin to visit weekly. At these visits, your doctor will continue to check weight, blood pressure, and baby measurements. You begin to see the doctor more frequently to screen for preterm labor and preeclampsia.

Hospital Paperwork

At this time, you should check to see if there is any specific hospital paperwork you need to fill out ahead of time, such as preregistration forms. Additionally, you may want to inquire about hospital policies for still photography and recording videos.

At thirty-five weeks, your doctor will begin to check your cervix. The cervix is the lowest part of your uterus. It is essentially the gate between your uterus and your vagina and has to open completely for the baby to be delivered. The cervix starts out the size and shape of a little, two-inch, white powdered donut and is located at the top of your vagina. The person checking your cervix inserts her finger(s) into the donut hole to determine your dilation, effacement, and station. If she cannot insert her finger at all into the donut, this means you are not dilated. If you are dilated, then she can also determine the effacement (thickness) and the station (height) of the cervix.

Effacement

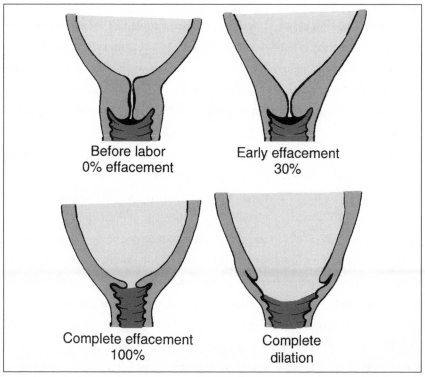

Before labor
0% effacement

Early effacement
30%

Complete effacement
100%

Complete
dilation

When we check the cervix, we feel for the amniotic membranes and usually baby's head as well. By feeling the size of the opening in the donut hole, we determine how many centimeters you are dilated. Dilation goes from zero (closed) to ten (no remaining cervix to be felt). The cervix starts as a "thick" donut, approximately three centimeters thick. It will slowly thin as you labor, until it is as thin as paper. So someone whose donut is only 1½ centimeters thick would be fifty percent effaced, and someone whose donut is paper-thin is one hundred percent effaced. The *station* is how high up the baby is, or rather how far into the vagina the doctor has to reach until she feels the head. This is a little tricky to determine. A baby who is very high is -3, and a baby who is visible at the labia is +3. So the station measurements go -3, -2, -1, 0, +1, +2, +3, then delivery. When the doctor checks your cervix and she says you are 1/50%/-3, that means your cervix is open one centimeter, it's half as thick as it was originally, and the baby is sitting high up in your vagina.

By checking your cervix, your doctor can make sure that the head is down and see whether the baby is in the correct position. As a general rule, most first-time moms will not dilate until closer to delivery, whereas women who have been pregnant before will begin to dilate a little earlier.

Your cervix is made out of very special skin, similar to your gums. So just like how your gums sometimes bleed when you floss or brush your teeth, your cervix will sometimes bleed after being checked. This isn't a "bad" thing, just a side effect of the increased blood flow to these organs in pregnancy.

You may also notice a change in your discharge as your cervix begins to dilate. Your cervix is made of glands that produce mucus; as it opens, it produces more mucus which results in an increased amount of discharge. Sometimes this increase in discharge will come out initially in a large amount. People like to refer to this as a "mucous plug." It often has the consistency of snot and will be tinged with blood. There is no need to take a picture of your mucous plug and text it to your doctor's cell phone! *This is gross, even for an OB*. There is also no need to call your doctor at 3 a.m. to let her know you lost your mucous plug. The passage of the mucous plug means that your body is preparing for labor, but it is not a guarantee that labor is coming very soon.

At your thirty-five-week visit, your doctor will perform a test to check for GBS (Group Beta Streptococcus). Different bacteria live in (colonize) the skin in different parts of your body. About fifteen percent of women have GBS bacteria in their vagina. This does not cause infection in the mom, but it can cause infection in the baby. The mom will have no symptoms from this colonization. She doesn't "catch" it from anywhere. It is just part of the normal bacteria that can live in the vagina. Since the baby's immune system is so weak at birth, and he spends so much time in the birth canal, he is more prone to infection. If your test comes back positive for GBS, then you will be treated with antibiotics during labor. Penicillin is the recommended treatment, so if you are allergic, remind your doctor at the time of this test. Colonization with GBS is transient. You may have it in one pregnancy, but not the next. That's why we wait until near delivery to screen for it.

Pain Management during Labor

This is probably one of the more stressful and debated topics of labor and delivery. Everyone likes to give you an opinion and a story, yet some people have very selective memories. "I had natural childbirth, and it didn't hurt at all!" Others will tell you their horror stories: "I was in labor for seven days and my epidural wore off and I felt *everything*!"

How you handle pain management during labor is your decision. Not your mom's, your sister's, or even your partner's (although you should probably involve him in the decision). It's something you both need to pray through and research. When you make up your mind, don't let other people's stories scare you or draw you into debate. It's perfectly normal to be scared. Really, every first-time mom is scared and intimidated by the labor process, no matter what her plan for pain control.

Epidural

An epidural is the most common form of pain management in the U.S. It works by giving the pain and numbing medicine directly into the space in your back where the nerves are located. The benefit of the epidural is that minimal pain medicine goes into your bloodstream, so neither you nor the baby is sedated by the epidural. An epidural has a very low rate of major complications.

If you are obese or have had back surgery, it may be more difficult for the epidural to be inserted. If you desire an epidural and have had back surgery before, you should probably meet with the anesthesiologist at your hospital before delivery so he or she can review your X-rays and see whether an epidural will be possible for you.

An epidural does not increase the rate of cesarean section, but it does decrease the intensity of contractions, which increases the need for Pitocin (a medication that induces labor contractions). Doctors and hospitals have different policies concerning when you can and cannot get an epidural. Some doctors will want you to be three or four centimeters dilated before you get it. Others allow you to get it upon arrival to the hospital. Once you get the epidural, you are confined to your bed and can no longer move around. One thought behind waiting for the epidural is to use the gravity of movement for as long as possible to help facilitate labor. At other centers, an epidural may not be available once you pass a certain dilation, such as eight centimeters. So, if you are planning to go natural and change your mind, you may not be able to get an epidural immediately.

It is recommended that the epidural be given at patient request. Sometimes this is not feasible (I have some patients request their epidural at their first pregnancy visit), so we have to take this on a case-by-case basis. Occasionally, the epidural will not work properly. The incidence of this is pretty rare, perhaps 1 in 500 births. You should expect to feel some sensation, even with a good epidural. You will still feel pressure and some discomfort. I am not saying this to scare you, but to prepare you that even with an epidural you will have some feeling during childbirth.

A *walking epidural* is where the anesthesiologist injects the pain medicine but not the numbing medicine. This allows you to walk around longer, but it does not offer enough relief for delivery. It does give you some added time to allow gravity to work in helping to bring the baby down further into your pelvis, but it doesn't deaden everything as fully as a regular epidural.

Intravenous Pain Medication

Pain medicine can be given through the IV; however, its effects are usually brief and can make you feel sedated. The IV medicine does cross the placenta, so we don't give it near delivery, since it can affect the baby's breathing. If someone is in early labor and is not yet ready for an epidural, then IV medicine can sometimes be given to lessen the intensity of the pain. This is not a great option for pain control near delivery, though.

Natural Childbirth Methods

If you desire natural childbirth, there are options that can help reduce your discomfort during labor. I recommend solid preparation before delivery by either reading books or attending classes. There are several tools that can help during natural childbirth. You should ask if your hospital has birthing balls or whether you need to bring your own. *Birthing balls* are exercise balls that can be used in early labor to help bring the baby into the pelvis. Some hospitals have birthing tubs or bathtubs in the room for relaxing during early labor. You may also want to bring a back massager for your husband to massage your lower back.

Natural versus Epidural

Natural		Epidural	
Pros	Cons	Pros	Cons

Movement
More effective pushing
Able to change
    positions
Not confined to bed
More control of body
	Pain
	Uncertainty
	Need for general
	    anesthesia if
	    emergent cesarean
	    section needed
		Pain controlled
		Less pain while
		    vaginal tear
		    is repaired
		Able to focus on
		    delivery and
		    not just pain
			Less urge to push
			Longer pushing stage
			Difficult to push
			    properly
			Unable to move
			    around
			Limited pushing
			    positions
			Need for Pitocin
			    increased

Preparing a Birth Plan

If you have specific things that are important to you during labor, I encourage you to write them down and discuss them with your doctor in the office, as well as with your labor nurse on arrival at the hospital. I find that a lot of birth plans can read like a hotel concierge request (e.g., make sure my room has comfortable pillows, a cot for my husband, and no noisy neighbors).

Alternately, sometimes women just point and click, printing things off the Internet without thinking about it. I once had a patient who included something I had never heard of on her birth plan. When I asked her what it meant and why it was important to her, she said, "I'm not sure, but the Web site said you should do it!" I do think it's a good idea to make a birth plan, as it allows you to think through all of the choices that will be presented to you when you go into labor. We've included a sample birth plan in the Appendix to get you started.

Some Considerations for Your Birth Plan

Natural childbirth, epidural ASAP, or labor as long as possible then epidural?

If you desire natural childbirth, then let that be the top item on your birth plan. Your doctor and nurse should work with you to achieve your goal. Honestly, there are some nurses who enjoy coaching natural childbirth more than others. So if you let the staff know up front, they can try to assign you the nurse that will work best with you.

If you want to labor for a while before you receive your epidural, you will also want to communicate that fully. Depending on how many other moms are in labor, it's possible you might have to wait a little while for the epidural (if everyone wants one at the same time). If you communicate with your nurse approximately when in labor you want your epidural, she will try to help you get it at the best time.

Music or quiet?

If you want to have specific music playing for delivery, you may want to start working on your playlist now. This is a good job for your husband. Some hospitals have sound systems, but for the most part, you will need to bring your own. This may seem like a trivial thing, but most people spend a lot of time in the delivery room, so you probably want to plan ahead for some entertainment.

Walk around in labor or stay in room?

If you desire to have natural childbirth, then you may want to walk during labor or move freely around the room. A lot of units will have mobile monitoring or, if the baby's heartbeat looks healthy, you can sometimes do intermittent monitoring. This involves the nurse listening to the heartbeat every ten to fifteen minutes versus being attached to a monitor.

Intravenous saline lock?

Most hospitals require that you have an IV in place in case of emergencies. You can request to have a heparin lock if you desire to move around. This means that you won't be attached to the IV pole and will be more mobile.

Watch delivery in mirror?

Some patients want to watch the birth in a mirror. Others find it helpful with pushing to watch the baby's head crown. Conversely, some don't want to know anything about what's going on in their "nether regions."

Hold baby immediately or nurses wipe him off first?

First off, don't feel like a bad mom if you want the baby wiped off before you hold him. They come out pretty bloody and gooey. If you do want to hold him right away, that's great, just let the doctors know.

Dad cut cord?

Most dads usually cut the cord, but if your husband is like mine—turning green at even the thought of blood—then you may want to have the doctor do this.

Who can be present at delivery?

Some hospitals limit the number of people that can be present for delivery, so you should find out in advance and decide whom you want present. This can be tricky at times, especially if both future grandmas want to be present, and the hospital limit is two people in the delivery room.

You may also want to think about who you want visiting while you are in labor. I'm amazed at the number of people who come visit women while they are in labor, but that is a personal decision. This is where you can use the hospital staff as the "bad guy." If you don't want to hurt the random visitor's feelings, you can have the nurses ask him or her politely to leave.

Breastfeed immediately or wait until after family visits?

It's important to try to breastfeed as soon as possible, but you also have to think about all the family in the waiting room waiting to see the baby. So, you should think through how you want to handle initial visitors and baby's feeding.

Doulas

Do you need a doula? Well, that depends. If you desire natural childbirth, then it is definitely something to consider, especially if your partner does not embrace the role of childbirth coach. A doula is a hired professional who will stay with you throughout your entire labor, providing emotional support and acting as a labor coach. Doulas are helpful with suggesting positions for labor and helping you enjoy the moment. There are also postpartum doulas who help with the postpartum transition and breastfeeding. For more information about doulas, check out www.dona.org.

Common Questions You May Have This Month

My breasts do not seem to have enlarged, and I haven't noticed any colostrum. Will I have trouble breastfeeding?

No. Neither the size of the breasts nor early breast discharge is indicative of your ability to fully breastfeed your baby.

Can you really tell with just an exam how dilated I am?

Yes. After lots of practice, doctors and labor nurses can very accurately assess the dilation of your cervix. My fingers are like calipers, accurate up to ten centimeters.

Do doctors know when women are going to go into labor?

No. We're not holding out on you, I promise. We can make an educated guess, but we have no way of knowing when you will go into labor. And, as my husband can attest, we also don't know how long your labor will last. (I'm often home much later than I initially tell him.)

How long will I stay in the hospital?

This will vary depending on the type of delivery and your preference. Usually, vaginal delivery is two days, whereas cesarean section is three to four days. Also, some states have specific laws requiring insurance to pay for a given amount of time in the hospital. Your doctor should be aware of any specific state laws that apply to this question.

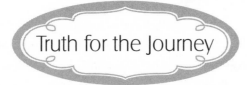

Truth for the Journey

But he said to me, 'My grace is sufficient for you, for my power
is made perfect in weakness.' Therefore I will boast all the more
gladly about my weaknesses, so that Christ's power may rest on me.
2 Corinthians 12:9

Seems like this verse has been ringing in my ears lately. I find myself saying it out loud several times a day. I cannot think of a more perfect time to memorize and recite this verse than in preparation for your labor. If this is your first baby, there is no way to know what your labor will be like. If this is your second or third or fourth child, there still is really no way to know exactly what the experience will hold, although you do have an idea of the pain involved. Either way, you will desperately need the grace and power of Christ to rest on you in that delivery room. There is no doubt about that!

Before you can even begin to think about all of the details of your labor, take some time to meditate on this verse and put your mind and heart at ease. Yes, this will likely be the hardest thing you have ever done in your life, but I guarantee you it will be the most rewarding as well. As long as you are prepared both mentally and spiritually for this experience, you will have the peace you need not just to get through it but to enjoy it as well.

When my husband and I were considering our options for labor and delivery, I asked him how he felt about the possibility of going through labor naturally and drug-free. His response surprised me. He told me he wanted the experience to be enjoyable. This was the day our first child would be born. He wanted to soak in every moment with peace and joy. He felt the best way to do that was to make sure I was as drugged as possible. I was torn as I thought through my options. My mother had me naturally. I wanted to prove I was as strong as she was; yet, after hearing this perspective from my husband, I knew I needed to take his request seriously. As it turned out, I ended up being induced due to last-minute complications. Natural labor would have been much harder with the intense contractions that came with induction. Our decision to receive an epidural was the right one for us for several reasons.

The important thing is that you carefully and prayerfully consider all of your options for labor and delivery. Don't feel like you have to go natural because your girlfriend did. Conversely, don't feel pressure to have an epidural because people say you are crazy for not having one. The decisions that come with this experience are very personal. Spend time praying together with your husband or family and go with your convictions. You will know what's right for you and your baby.

Make sure to plan a last-minute pedicure. You get a great massage on your swollen legs and feet, and then you have pretty toes for the big day! And let's face it. It may be the last time you get to pamper yourself for quite a while. Abi, 36, mother of two

Pediatric Provider Checklist

☐ Do they accept my insurance?

☐ Are the office hours convenient? (This is especially important for working moms.)

☐ Is the location convenient?

☐ Will I talk to the doctor or a nurse if I call with non-emergency questions?

☐ Is this doctor affiliated with the hospital where I will deliver?

☐ What is their philosophy on breastfeeding versus bottle-feeding?

☐ What is their philosophy on scheduling? Getting baby to sleep?

☐ What is their philosophy on immunizations? What if I want to alter the normal schedule for my child?

Now is the time you may want to begin researching and interviewing pediatricians (if you haven't already). The things to consider when choosing a pediatrician are similar to those Dr. Rupe discussed in regard to choosing an OB—making sure they take your insurance and have a clean and efficient office, for example. In addition, there are several other factors to think about before committing to a pediatric physician. It may help to make an appointment to interview or at least meet a few doctors in your area. We have included a list of questions to ask when considering a pediatrician. You may have additional items to add to this list based on your personal preferences and convictions about the care of your baby.

The best recommendation you can receive for a doctor may be from a friend or family member who shares your philosophies on issues such as feeding and immunizations. Ask your girlfriends or co-workers who they use and why. In the end, it is most important that you have a pediatrician with whom you feel comfortable and who won't make you feel stupid for asking all of the normal first-time mom questions.

Postpartum Care

This might be a good time to read ahead to Chapter Eleven where we discuss postpartum care. You can never overprepare yourself for what you may experience after your baby's birth. Take a few moments to review the information on the physical and emotional needs you will have after delivery. Talk about them with your spouse or family so you can best prepare for the road ahead.

I hope that by now you have developed a great respect for your OB. As you look toward your delivery date, don't be afraid to ask lots of questions, but remember that once you are in the midst of working to help your little one enter this world, you have to trust your doctor. As I said earlier, there is no way to know what is going to happen on delivery day. Your doctor is trained and knows what to do in every situation. If you don't feel now that you would let your doctor do whatever she thought necessary to protect you and your baby, then maybe you should find a new OB, quickly!

No matter what happens in that delivery room, remember that God's grace is sufficient for you. Whether you choose to play soothing worship music as you labor or simply pray through the experience, invite Christ's power to rest on you as you contend with the pain and discomfort to welcome your baby into the world.

Prayer Concerns

Final stages of baby's growth and development

Mommy's comfort

Labor and delivery decisions

Doctor's wisdom

Delivery day!

A Prayer for This Month

Dear Lord,

I admit that I am a bit scared about the delivery. I know that you created my body to bring life into this world. I trust that you will see it to completion until I am holding my baby in my arms. Give us wisdom, Lord, as we decide what measures to take during labor. May your power rest on me as I take part in an amazing miracle. Your grace is sufficient. I thank you for it. Amen.

Write a prayer here for your own personal journey.

_____

_____

_____

_____

_____

Journal

Record your thoughts and your fears here. It is important to acknowledge every thought and feeling you are experiencing. The main thing is to get them out in the open, and if they do not line up with the truth or the faith that you possess, then get rid of those burdens by giving them over to your Pregnancy Companion.

_____

_____

_____

_____

_____

Chapter Nine

Will I Ever Feel Ready for This?
Weeks 36 to 40

Key Bible Verse

*Let us not become weary in doing good, for at the proper
time we will reap a harvest if we do not give up.*

Galatians 6:9

Baby Stats

Your baby is full term starting at thirty-seven weeks! The average baby is around
7½ pounds and nineteen inches long at birth, but this is only the average. All systems should be fully developed. He's getting cramped in his environment though,
so you may feel his movements changing a bit; instead of the big kicks and flips,
now he's mainly wiggles.

Mommy Stats

I will admit something in this book. When I start to enter a patient's room for an
office visit and notice that she is term (after thirty-seven weeks), I will stop to take
a breath and prepare myself. I am not usually met with many smiles when I open
that door. There are some pretty miserable pregnant women out there who can
be very vocal. When I start with the usual "How are you doing?" I am often met
with some seriously evil looks. This tends to be a time of significant discomfort.
You hurt. You contract. You are swollen. And if one more person asks when you're

due, you are likely to resort to physical violence. Oh, wait, you're too big for physical violence!

In all seriousness, this is one of the most challenging times in pregnancy, certainly not for all women but for a significant majority. At this point, you have likely gained twenty-five to thirty pounds, and it's probably getting difficult to tie your shoes. Your body is full of hormones as it prepares for delivery. You have a fifty percent increase in blood volume by this point, and your heart is pumping faster than normal. You may also begin to feel more tired with activity. This is due to a combination of hormones and the physical space occupied by the baby pushing up on your lungs. Rest assured that some of your discomfort will soon be resolved . . . although I can't promise more sleep.

Symptom Checker

- ☐ Constipation or hemorrhoids
- ☐ Heartburn
- ☐ Backaches
- ☐ Enlarged breasts
- ☐ Swelling
- ☐ Leg cramps
- ☐ Frequent urination
- ☐ Colostrum
- ☐ Bleeding gums
- ☐ Shortness of breath
- ☐ Sleeplessness
- ☐ Clumsiness
- ☐ Fetal movement
- ☐ Occasional contractions

Frequent urination. You will most likely continue to experience frequent urination. This is caused by the giant head sitting on your bladder. Pressure is normal; however, if you have burning or pain when you urinate, notify your doctor, as this could signal an infection.

Sleeplessness. Sleep becomes increasingly difficult toward the end of pregnancy. We often joke that this is to get you ready for the sleepless nights you'll have with your newborn. It is actually because it is difficult to get comfortable during the last couple of weeks. Some women find it easier to sleep in a recliner. Most women have to get up several times at night to urinate, and it can be difficult to fall back to sleep. The baby is often more active at night as well. Drinking herbal tea and relaxing in a warm bath can help improve your sleep. If this still doesn't work, ask your doctor if an over-the-counter sleep aid would be safe for you.

Contractions. Usually contractions will increase, as well as the feeling of pressure, when baby "drops" (begins to descend into the birth canal). This pressure can be rather constant and feel like there is a bowling ball between your legs, because essentially there is! The contractions may wax and wane over the next few weeks, but as a general rule, you want to call the doctor when they are painful and five minutes apart.

Expectations for This Month's Visit

You will be visiting your doctor weekly at this point. This is so she can assess for signs of labor and look for complications such as preeclampsia. Your doctor will continue to check your cervix, weight, and blood pressure. Some women gain several pounds a week in the last few weeks of pregnancy. This is usually more related to fluid retention and swelling than actual weight gain, which means it should go away as quickly as it came once the baby is born.

Bleeding. You may experience a small amount of bleeding after cervical exams. By this I mean when you wipe, you may notice streaks of blood on the tissue. If you experience any bleeding more than this, you should call your doctor.

Decreased movement. Your biggest reassurance on a day-to-day basis that your baby is healthy is his movement. You must continue to do your kick counts every day. He should be moving at least six times an hour once a day. If during the hour that you are counting, you do not feel six movements, lie down, drink some juice, and then recount during the next hour. If you still don't get six movements, call your doctor immediately.

Water breaking. Call your doctor if your water breaks. How do you know if your water broke? In most instances, it is obvious: fluid goes everywhere. I have met a lot of women who live in fear of their water breaking in strange places. They put shower curtains over their car upholstery "just in case" it breaks in the car, so it doesn't ruin their leather. Only about five percent of women will have their water break before the onset of labor.

Sometimes the leaking of fluid is not a big gush but rather a trickle. This can make it trickier. If you feel increased moisture and you're not sure if it's discharge from that pesky cervix, urine from your leaking bladder, or actually amniotic fluid, then here's a trick you can try: fully empty your bladder, dry your bottom completely with a towel, lay down for thirty minutes, and then sit up to see if fluid comes out. If it does, then this is most likely your water breaking. If everything remains dry, then it was probably just your leaky bladder. Obviously, if you are undecided, notify your doctor so she can check things out. Your amniotic fluid is clear and odorless and will usually continue to come out steadily.

Contractions. Your uterus is made of muscle. A labor contraction is literally a contraction of that muscle. It should feel like a painful tightening. Moms can get frustrated in the final weeks of pregnancy because they often have contractions, and it can sometimes be difficult to determine whether the contractions are "real" or not. True labor contractions are increasingly painful and regular. They don't go away; they continue to get more intense. You should time from the beginning of one contraction until the beginning of the next. When they are five minutes apart for an hour and painful, you should call your doctor about coming in. If this is not your first baby and you have been dilated in the office, or if you live a long way from the hospital, then your doctor may want you to call earlier.

Induction

I find a lot of women at this stage of pregnancy begging for induction of labor. Sometimes it's well beyond normal begging, more like "get this baby out of me or I might hurt you" kind of begging. *Induction* is when medications are given to start your labor. The medicines given will depend on the dilation of your cervix. If your cervix is closed, your body will need more help with the process. Either a medication called Cervidil or Cytotec is given the evening before the planned induction. These medications are topical medications placed in the vagina to help your cervix soften and prepare for labor. The next morning, Pitocin is begun to give you contractions.

Pitocin

Pitocin is an analogue of the hormone oxytocin that was first synthesized in the 1950s.[1] Oxytocin is a hormone produced by the brain that travels to the uterus and tells it to contract. Pitocin can be used to help increase the strength of contractions in women whose labor has slowed down (augmentation) or to help start labor (induction). It is given as an intravenous drip. The purpose of giving Pitocin is to help prevent cesarean sections, especially when a woman's labor has stalled. The intensity of contractions produced by Pitocin can sometimes be perceived as more painful than spontaneous labor. Also, the fetal heart rate is monitored closely while a woman is on Pitocin to make sure the contractions aren't too close together, which can cause the heart rate to drop. This means that she will need continuous monitoring and may not be able to move around as much in labor.

Induction is not without risks. The main risk of induction is cesarean section. The risk of cesarean section is increased by fifteen percent if you are having your first baby, and you are not very dilated at the time of induction. If you are having your second baby and are already dilated, the increased risk is not as large at three percent, but risk is still present. Induction can also be more painful than spontaneous labor, since the contractions become more intense more quickly. Rest assured, these intense contractions do not hurt the baby. With your first pregnancy especially, you want to avoid induction if possible. However, there are several medical reasons for induction.

One of the more common complications that can lead to induction is preeclampsia. This complication is more common with first pregnancies. With this condition, the blood pressure continues to elevate more and more until the baby is delivered. It is often preferable to induce labor once the baby is mature enough rather than wait, which could lead to more severe complications. Other reasons for induction include diabetes, low amniotic fluid, and other medical issues.

So while we don't want to induce labor early without good cause, there does come a point where "enough's enough." If you are past your due date, your doctor may discuss induction with you. Studies show a slightly increased risk of stillbirth after forty-one weeks. After forty-two weeks, there is a significantly increased risk of stillbirth. The risk of stillbirth goes from 1 per 1,000 at forty-one weeks to 3 per 1,000 at forty-two weeks.[2] So somewhere between forty-one and forty-two weeks, your doctor will most likely recommend induction.

Fear of having a big baby is not reason enough to induce. When we are watching a patient closely to make sure her baby doesn't get too big, she will often ask to be induced. While it seems to make sense to have the baby early so he is not too large, studies show that although the baby born early may be smaller, the risk of cesarean section for these deliveries is higher due to the fact that baby simply isn't ready to come out.

For some women, induction may include lower risk—if it's a second or third baby and if she is already a couple centimeters dilated. If she has family that needs to come in from out of town to keep her kids or other issues pressing, it is reasonable to consider induction for social reasons. On the other hand, a first-time mom who is not dilated at all and is basically just tired of being pregnant is probably not the best candidate for an induction. If you are planning natural childbirth, you will likely want to avoid induction unless medically necessary, because induction is generally more painful than natural labor.

How to Bring On Labor

So what's a miserable pregnant girl to do, doc, since you won't induce me? Eat eggplant? Walk for miles? There are a couple of things that have been shown to help bring on labor. The first is . . . actually how you got here in the first place: sex. The prostaglandins in semen have been shown to help increase contractions. So while you may not be feeling your most amorous right now, having intercourse may help get things headed in the right direction.

The other thing that can help bring on labor is having your doctor strip your membranes. This is similar to having your cervix checked, but slightly more painful. Remember the analogy of the donut (see Chapter Eight)? To strip the membranes, your doctor inserts her finger all the way through the donut hole (the opening in the cervix) and makes a circular motion between the uterus and the bag of water. This action helps the uterus release proteins that increase contractions.

Other things like walking and eating spicy food are thought to be helpful, but they have not been proven scientifically. I would avoid herbal supplements in an attempt to bring on labor because their safety has not yet been established.

Full Term Baby Near Delivery

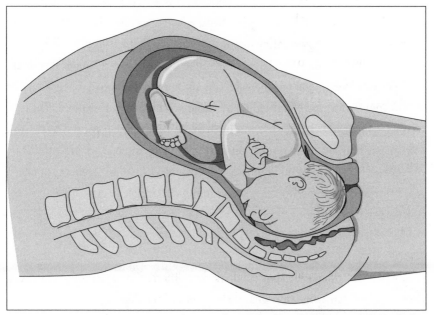

© 2010 Wolters Kluwer Health | Lippincott Williams and Wilkins

Labor and Delivery

The day is finally here. Your contractions are painful and coming five minutes apart, and you just called the doctor and she said "come on in." The adventure is truly beginning. You most likely have many hours ahead of you, so despite what happens on TV shows, you do not need to speed excessively to the hospital. Your husband will probably be nervous and preoccupied; don't add driving ninety miles an hour to your travel hazards.

Hopefully you have preregistered and know where you're heading in the hospital. If not, just go anywhere in the hospital, and someone will point you quickly to labor and delivery. Pretty much everyone in the hospital except OBs and labor nurses are scared of pregnant women, so they want you to get to the proper place as soon as possible. Nobody wants to deliver a baby in the elevator. If you have already submitted your insurance paperwork, then the admission process takes just a few minutes. They may have you sign some forms and then get you to labor and delivery, where the nurses will finish your admission process. Everyone admitted to the hospital, no matter what the reason, gets asked a zillion questions that are standard for the hospital or state. Cooperating may not be pleasant, but it will speed things up.

After all the endless questions, the nurse will start your IV, and if you are GBS positive (see Chapter Eight), she will start your antibiotics. Then after she checks your cervix, you can decide if and when you want your epidural. This will be the time that you can go over your birth plan with the nurse. Most nurses work shifts, so depending on what time you deliver, you may end up with more than one nurse. There may also be nursing assistants around to help with delivery or charting. If you have very specific requests on your birth plan, it's a good idea to review it with each new nurse.

Labor

Now comes the fun part. Labor can look very different for different people. As a general rule, labor with your second child goes faster than with your first. Early labor or "latent labor"—from one to four centimeters dilation—can take anywhere from two to twenty-four hours. Active labor is from four to ten centimeters, and this usually progresses more quickly, with dilation increasing one to two centimeters per hour.

Stages of Labor

First Baby

	Average	Abnormal
Latent labor 0–4 cm	< 20 hours	> 20 hours
Active labor 4–10 cm	1.2 cm per hour dilation	No dilation in 2 hours
Pushing with epidural	70 min	> 3 hours
Pushing without epidural	50 min	> 2 hours

Subsequent Babies

	Average	Abnormal
Latent labor 0–4 cm	< 12 hours	> 12 hours
Active labor 4–10 cm	1.5 cm per hour dilation	No dilation in 2 hours
Pushing with epidural	50 min	> 2 hours
Pushing without epidural	20 min	> 1 hour

If you have an epidural, you may want to watch TV or read books while you are in labor. If you are choosing natural childbirth, you will at this point be using your relaxation techniques. Normally, the doctor or nurses will check your cervix every two hours to make sure you are making progress and your cervix is continuing to dilate. If your labor begins to stall, the doctor may choose to start Pitocin, which increases the strength of your contractions. An internal monitor might be placed to measure the exact strength of your contractions.

Pushing

Once you reach dilation of ten centimeters, it is time to push. If you have an epidural, it's usually easier to push while lying on your back with both legs pulled back. Often your husband will help hold up one of your legs, and the nurses will hold the other. If you are choosing natural childbirth, you can usually push in whatever position feels most comfortable. Like most parts of labor, the amount of pushing varies greatly and is usually much less with your second child. With an epidural, you usually do not feel the sensation to push as strongly, so you often have to push longer. The average time of pushing with a first baby and an epidural is about an hour.

Delivery

I have delivered over a thousand babies, but still each one is a miracle. After delivery, you can often hold the baby right away if he is healthy. Moms often spend lots of time wondering what their baby will look like and dreaming about that first moment of seeing him.

Newborn babies are usually slimy, bloody, and blue. If you deliver vaginally, he could have a large cone head. So if your first instinct when you see your newborn is not to smother him with kisses, that is OK. The nurses will dry him off with a blanket, which will stimulate him to cry. When he is clean and pink, he will begin to look more like the baby you've been imagining. If you would like your delivery recorded or photographed, you should check beforehand to see if hospital policy will allow it.

Leakage. Let's talk a little bit about bodily fluids. During delivery, things happen that you don't necessarily anticipate. Like poop. A large majority of women poop while they are pushing *and that is normal*. The muscles that you use when you are pushing are the same ones you use to poop, so pooping is actually a sign that you are pushing correctly. Several of you just put this book down and made a gagging noise to the person sitting in the room with you. But the doctors and nurses who work labor and delivery are quite prepared for it and not disturbed by it at all.

After your water breaks you will continue to leak fluid, so you will have the constant sensation that you are peeing on yourself. You will be given pads to wear or place under you. You do actually pee with pushing sometimes as well, and this is also OK. Other fluids including mucus and blood will come out vaginally during labor. Vomiting is also common during labor. Not all labors will have all these things happen, but they are all very common and you need not feel embarrassed if they happen to you.

Vacuum and forceps. Sometimes it becomes necessary to deliver the baby very quickly. If the baby's heartbeat begins to drop, it can be a sign that he's not getting enough oxygen, and your doctor will begin to evaluate which is the quickest and safest way to deliver the baby. Once the baby is visible on the perineum, it's safer to deliver by vacuum or forceps than by cesarean section. If the heart rate drops and the mom can't push the baby out, the next step will be for the doctor to help facilitate delivery. The vacuum applies suction to the top of the head. It is shaped like a large disk. Forceps look like large spoons that go on the sides of the baby's head so that the doctor can apply traction to help guide the baby out.

I often have women tell me they don't want me to use a vacuum or forceps no matter what—they just want a C-section. I actually don't want to ever have to use forceps. I would love for all babies to pop right out and never have their heart rate drop. The truth is that the heart rate does drop at times, and there are a few specific instances where a vacuum or forceps is much safer for you and the baby. The idea of a vacuum or forceps delivery is scary, as can be the mere sight of forceps. This is where it becomes important to have a doctor that you can trust to make the right decision for you and your baby.

Episiotomy. An episiotomy is when the doctor makes an incision in the perineum (skin between the vagina and rectum) to allow more room for the baby to come out. Originally, episiotomy was performed to help prevent tearing, which was thought to cause more significant damage. Newer studies have shown this is not the case and that episiotomies can lead to worse tearing, so they are performed less routinely than in the past. If the baby is suspected to be very big or if the heart rate has dropped, an episiotomy might still be necessary.

The amount of tearing with delivery is rated on a scale from one to four. A level one tear involves just the superficial skin in the vagina, whereas a level four tear is when the skin tears all the way through into the rectum. Level one and two tears are the most common and usually heal within a couple of weeks. Level three and four tears are more rare, occurring in less than two percent of deliveries, thankfully. These tears do take longer to heal and are associated with more pain after delivery. They will get better with time, and pain medication can be taken for the discomfort.

Cesarean Section

There are a lot of emotions that are associated with even the word *C-section*. I find that sometimes women feel as though it is a personal failure if they need a C-section. This is simply not true! This is another area where people like to tell you their horror stories or give you their unsolicited opinions. Your goal is to have a healthy baby, first and foremost. My hope is that everyone's delivery goes smoothly and vaginally, but that is not always possible. I hope the following section will prepare you for what to expect should you need a C-section and to fully walk in as much peace as possible through that process.

A few reasons for doing a C-section instead of even trying labor are placenta previa, breech presentation, or a baby thought to be too large (usually over ten pounds). In these instances, the doctor will usually schedule a C-section for somewhere between thirty-nine and forty weeks. If you were to go into labor before the scheduled time, the doctor would do a C-section when labor was confirmed. Knowing in advance that you are having a C-section can be good and bad. You can prepare yourself for what to expect, but there is also a certain amount of fear that goes with having surgery. Combined with all the unknowns of having a baby, this can be a lot to process. Patients having a C-section without being in labor first usually have an easier recovery and less risk for complications.

The most common reasons to move from a vaginal delivery to a C-section are if your cervix stops dilating or the baby's heart rate begins to drop, and he shows signs that he may not be getting enough oxygen. If your cervix stops dilating, this could be a sign that the baby is too big or your pelvis is too small. Once you pass four centimeters, if your cervix goes more than two or three hours without dilating, your doctor may recommend a C-section. If the heart rate begins to show signs of decreased oxygen, this can sometimes lead to an emergency C-section. Emergency C-sections are rare, but when they happen there's a lot of commotion and not a lot of time to explain everything fully. If the baby is in trouble, time is of the essence, so the staff is going to get you to the operating room as quickly as possible.

Having a C-section is intimidating because it's such a huge mystery. The average person has never even been in an operating room before, at least not awake. One of the biggest fears people have associated with surgery is that they will have pain. Anesthesia doctors will make sure you are comfortable before they start the procedure. If the decision is made to perform a C-section and you have an epidural already in place, you will be given a larger dose of medicine through it. The nurses will shave your lower abdomen and put a catheter in your bladder. You will also be given a dose of antibiotics to help prevent infection from surgery.

The nurses will roll your bed into the OR, which is a large, cold, brightly-lit room where everyone is scuttling around wearing masks. Your husband will usually stay outside the door until the staff has everything set up. The nurse will clean your belly with a sterile soap, then sterile drapes will be placed over you. The drape is often very close to your face, so if you tend to be claustrophobic, just request that they readjust the drape. Your husband will then join you as they start the procedure.

The sensation is similar to when you go to the dentist. You should be completely numb and not feel any pain, but you will occasionally feel some pulling sensation or pressure. You will hear lots of different noises. When the baby is born, you may feel some pressure sensations on your belly. Oftentimes, you will be able to see the baby shortly after birth. After the baby is out, the anesthesiologist may put medicine in the IV to help you relax if needed. After the procedure, the nurse will roll you to a recovery room, where you will be able to nurse and hold your little bundle of joy.

Vaginal Birth after Cesarean Section (VBAC)

If your first delivery was a cesarean section, now is the time to consider whether you want to try a vaginal delivery or whether you prefer a repeat cesarean section. Until the 1980s, the medical recommendation was that once you had a C-section, you should have a C-section for any later pregnancies. This was due to the risk of the uterine scar breaking open while a mom was in labor. In the 80s and 90s, studies were done showing that in certain circumstances it was safe to have a vaginal delivery after C-section. Risk of the uterus breaking open was found to be less than one percent in women who were proper candidates and went into labor on their own.

Moms often ask me which is better and safer for their baby. This question is difficult to answer and needs to be individualized to the patient. A VBAC that results in a successful vaginal delivery without problems is always the best-case scenario. The problem is that an attempted VBAC resulting in an emergency C-section delivery during labor is the worst. There is not a perfect way to know who will have to have an emergency C-section and who will have the successful vaginal delivery.

When an emergency C-section is done on someone who has already had a C-section, it makes it more difficult to get the baby out of the mom quickly and safely due to scar tissue. Also, when a uterine rupture happens (less than one percent of VBAC deliveries), it can be a truly emergent event, possibly resulting in severe hemorrhage in the mom, neurological injury in the baby, and emergency hysterectomy. The baby can also be deprived of oxygen, which can lead to brain damage or death. Having multiple C-sections is not without complication either; with each additional C-section, the risk of scar tissue and bladder damage increases. Due to liability risk or lack of anesthesia availability, VBACs are not offered in some areas of the country.

There are guidelines to consider and discuss with your doctor when considering VBAC. If you had a previous vaginal delivery and then a C-section, your risk of rupture is lower and your chance of successful VBAC is higher. If you desire to have more than three children, you might consider VBAC more strongly because the risk associated with C-sections increases after your third C-section. If it is very important to you to experience a vaginal delivery, and the reasons for your first C-section were unique (such as your first baby was breech), then you should strongly consider VBAC—in that instance, your success rate is around seventy-five percent. However, if the reason for getting a previous C-section cannot be changed, such as your pelvic bones were too small for a normal-sized baby to pass through, then the likelihood of the next normal-sized baby passing through them is low, and perhaps the risk of the complications would not be worth it.

The following is a list of general guidelines for VBAC indications:

- Hospital equipped to care for VBAC patients
  - In-house anesthesiology
  - In-house OB/GYN
  - Ability to quickly perform a C-section
- Pelvic bones large enough for baby to pass through
- Spontaneous labor (no induction)
- One or two previous C-sections
- Normal previous C-section (not a "classical" where the scar is vertical on the uterus)
- Baby is not too big

So a successful VBAC is always the best-case scenario, but a labor that has to be converted to a repeat C-section can increase the risk of complications in mom and baby. There is no way to know before labor whose VBAC will be successful. Discuss your specific situation with your doctor to make the best decision for you and your baby.

Managing Expectations

Moms spend their whole pregnancy dreaming about delivery and picturing how it is going to play out. While this is fun to do at times, it can also lead to unrealistic expectations. Your delivery may not go according to plan. You may not feel exactly how you think you are going to feel when you see your baby for the first time. Your husband may not immediately cry tears of joy. Your first words when seeing your baby might be "EWW!" I've had a few people say something like this and then apologize to me for days that this was their reaction. Try not to script out your labor and delivery. Your team of doctors and nurses want things to go according to plan, but sometimes unforeseen complications happen. Be ready, but also be ready for anything. Ask the Lord to cover you and give you peace no matter how the day (or night) goes.

The Doctor's POV: Labor and Delivery

At thirty-two weeks, I learned that my son was breech, so I knew I would be having a cesarean section. There is a procedure called a *version*, where the doctor can attempt to flip the baby around; however, this is something I didn't feel comfortable trying. I was in my OB/GYN residency training during my pregnancy, which was challenging, since I often worked eighty hours a week, twelve to fourteen hours a day. I had scheduled my C-section for thirty-nine weeks, and my parents had their plane tickets to come out. Everything was all planned out.

A few days before the big day, I woke up feeling even more tired than normal. I was assisting with several surgeries that day, and it was during the first case that the headache started. Then during the second case, I started seeing little spots. I stopped by labor and delivery after the case, and my blood pressure was through the roof. The urine dip (yes, I dipped my own urine) was a pretty shade of purple protein.

Luckily, one of my fellow residents and close friends observed these things and called my doctor. I had no insight. Intellectually, I realized I had preeclampsia, but it didn't compute emotionally. It was strange. I was flabbergasted that things would happen out of order. My baby was to be born on Saturday. I realized I was terrified of the unknown despite performing hundreds of C-sections myself. Several blubbering phone calls later, they set me up for delivery.

My husband and four friends who were fellow residents were there to support me. The whole room cheered when my son was born. "It's a boy!" someone said. They announced it over the loudspeaker in the labor and delivery wing, too. I remember them holding him up over the blue sheet, and I thought they should really get him to the warmer. Myself, my husband, and my friends (who were running various video cameras) were all crying and cheering. It was an amazing day. I had practically lived at this hospital for three years, so it was awesome to have my baby among family.

The Patient's POV: Labor and Delivery

I was induced at 37½ weeks because we discovered a few days before that I had a kidney stone. I began to feel horrible pain and, being a first-time mom, I thought I might be going into labor. My co-worker took me to see Dr. Rupe, and she quickly determined the pain was not labor but instead a pesky stone. I was admitted to the hospital where I spent two nights after having a stint inserted in my ureter. As if the last stages of pregnancy aren't uncomfortable enough, try walking around feeling like you have to pee 24/7, with a full-term baby pressing on your bladder. It was not fun! Dr. Rupe, the high-risk specialist, and the urologist decided that delivery was indicated, so we scheduled an induction. Have I mentioned that I love Dr. Rupe?

As far as inductions go, mine was a pretty textbook experience. We arrived at the hospital around 7 A.M. By 7:30, I was hooked up to an IV and had started my Pitocin. When I was four centimeters dilated, Dr. Rupe broke my water. She did this by inserting an instrument that looked like a huge knitting needle inside me. Moments later, I felt a gush of fluid. I had told Dr. Rupe I wanted to experience as much natural labor as possible, so we waited a bit after breaking my water to start the epidural. Contractions tend to strengthen after your water breaks, so by that time I was really feeling my labor. I enjoyed being able to experience some of the pain that comes with having a baby. I suppose I was simply curious to know what all the fuss is about.

The anesthesiologist had to do my epidural twice because the first time it didn't take. Although it was tough remaining still in the middle of contractions for two epidural needles, once it was successfully in, I was able to lay back and relax through the hardest part of my labor.

After a few hours of relaxation, I began to experience severe pressure in my rectal region. Girls, this was not something I was prepared for. I literally felt like my baby girl wanted to exit the back door instead of the front. I'm still not sure why I felt this type of discomfort, since most of the women I talked to had not. It's important to remember that you may feel some level of pain even with an epidural. Everybody is different, so there's no way to know for sure how you will respond.

I was able to work through the pain with focused breathing (and a little crying) until it was time to push. I began pushing at 7:15 P.M., roughly twelve hours after we started the induction process. Hope was born at 8:05 P.M. after the most difficult, yet rewarding physical experience of my life. Dr. Rupe, the nurses, my husband, and my mother were all there to coach me through to the end. I will never forget the amazing feeling that came with seeing my little girl for the first time. It was well worth the work and the wait!

Common Questions You May Have This Month

What if I go into labor and don't know it?
I get this question a lot, but I have never had it happen in my practice. Labor is quite painful and usually obvious. If your doctor finds that you are starting to dilate a lot during one of your weekly office visits, she may instruct you to come to the hospital when you begin experiencing minimal discomfort.

I have a history of herpes. Does this mean I'll need a C-section?
If you have a herpes outbreak at the time of delivery, then yes, you will need a C-section. If you have a history of herpes (up to fifteen percent of the population

does), then you need to be placed on suppressive medication in the last month of pregnancy to help prevent an outbreak at the time of delivery. As long as there is no outbreak, then you can have a vaginal delivery.

My baby seems to have the hiccups all the time. Is that normal?
Yes. Hiccups are a sign of a very healthy baby.

I have HPV. Will this affect my delivery?
No. HPV is a sexually transmitted virus that as many as seventy percent of women will contract in their twenties. It can cause abnormal Pap smears or genital warts. It does not have any effect on pregnancy or delivery, even if you have a genital wart at the time of delivery.

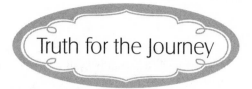

Truth for the Journey

Let us not become weary in doing good, for at the
proper time we will reap a harvest if we do not give up.
Galatians 6:9

Is it starting to sink in? The thought that you are very close to pushing a watermelon out of a hole the size of a kiwi, that is. Your impending labor may be at the forefront of your mind right now, and that is to be expected, especially if this is your first baby. One of my favorite things about Dr. Rupe as an obstetrician is that she is completely no-nonsense. She's delivered over a thousand babies, and she's just about seen it all. I can assure you that the information and advice she's given you in this chapter is just about all you'll need to know if you are moving toward a textbook-type birth. Every once in a while, nature throws a curveball, though, so make sure to discuss any questions or concerns with your doctor as soon as you get the chance.

I chose this month's key Bible verse because it's one that has always encouraged me to keep going when I wanted to give up. At this point, you may be experiencing discomfort, sleepless nights, and apprehensive thoughts of delivering this child (let alone raising him!). We are reminded in Galatians 6:9 that we cannot let ourselves become weary. What you are enduring right now will lead to something so wonderful and good. At the proper time—that moment when your little one decides to grace the world—you will reap a harvest that will be well worth the work and the wait.

I had very clear ideas of how I thought my pregnancy and the birthing process should be. When the big day arrived, my body and my daughter had other ideas. My natural labor became excruciating due to back labor pain and because I never fully dilated. This caused me to have an emergency C-section. I was devastated. But when she came out at a surprising and whopping ten pounds, eleven ounces, I was overwhelmed with how God protected me and my daughter. I learned an early and valuable lesson about letting go and not being so structured. Kris, 37, mother of one

So don't give up now. You are so close! Obviously, you can't just "give up" with a life still physically growing inside your belly. But I don't want you to give up mentally or emotionally, either. Keep your head and your heart in this process as you near its completion. You will not believe the work that the Lord can do in you during these last few weeks. As we've said before, you are personally taking part in one of the most amazing miracles. This might just be the best time in your life to feel the greatness of God all over you.

You may feel overwhelmed by the many factors to consider for your birthing process. Hopefully you have spent some time thinking and praying over them. You should also realize that some of these things may be out of your control during labor and delivery. Be careful not to spend too much time scripting how you want your experience to go, as you will more than likely be disappointed. I'm not saying you can't plan for the way you would like labor to go. You simply need to understand that it may not go that way. As we've said before, what matters most in the moment is that mommy and baby are safe and healthy. Whatever it takes to reach that end result will be the correct course of action.

You've spent time discussing your options with your spouse or family, and now I want you to stop and pray and ask God to guide you through this process. The most important preparation you can make going into your labor is to be ready for anything. The best ways for you to do this are to be fully surrendered to the Lord through prayer and to have complete trust in your doctor. Are you there yet? Great. Now we can do some more planning.

If you are scheduled for an induction or C-section, you will be able to plan for your baby's upcoming birthday. Packing beforehand and arranging childcare (if needed) will be easy if you know the exact day of your little one's arrival. If you are simply waiting for those contractions to clue you in to his coming, try to plan as much as possible, as being prepared will alleviate any unneeded stress in the last few weeks of your pregnancy.

As you walk through the remaining weeks of your pregnancy, I pray that you will have an abundance of strength and joy. So many women go through the home stretch uncomfortable, irritable, and miserable. This does not have to be the case for you. Continue to tap into the grace of God that is available to you as you ask him for it. Do not become weary as you continue this good work. Your harvest is just around the corner.

After nine months of dreams and visions about your little one, you will discover the fascinating miracle God has created just for you on the day of their birth. The phrase, "love at first sight" could only have been originated for a time such as this. Gigi, 62, mother of three, grandmother of three

When the amazing day of your child's birth finally arrives, I encourage you to ask the Creator of life to be with you in every moment. A heart full of peace will be the most inviting place for him to dwell, so spend ample time with your spouse or family in prayer as you move toward the big day. I can't think of a better Companion for the birthing process than the One who is responsible for the miracle of life. He will be with you as you labor, and his heart will leap for joy with yours as your little one is placed in your arms.

Pre-Labor Checklist

☐ Hospital bag packed.

☐ Car seat installed. Check out www.seatcheck.org or the National Highway Traffic Safety Administration Web site to make sure your seat is properly installed in your car.

☐ Childcare options arranged. It is important to have a few friends or family members on standby, since their availability will depend on what day you go into labor.

☐ Meals planned. Someone will probably offer to help with meals after your delivery. Let them! At least ask your mom or sister or best friend to stock your fridge and pantry with groceries while you are in the hospital. This way, you'll have fresh food upon your return home.

☐ Playlist created. If you would like to listen to music during your labor, plan ahead so you can have your favorite tunes collected on CD or an MP3 player.

Hospital Bag Checklist

- ☐ Copy of your birth plan
- ☐ Health insurance cards or documents
- ☐ Comfortable pajamas (you should be able to wear these after labor and delivery)
- ☐ Slippers
- ☐ Your favorite pillow
- ☐ Underwear
- ☐ Socks (the delivery room may be cold)
- ☐ Personal hygiene items (if you can, a shower after delivery will feel great)
- ☐ Makeup you simply can't live without
- ☐ Baby's going home outfit
- ☐ Mommy's going home outfit
- ☐ Baby blanket
- ☐ Breastfeeding supplies and perhaps a book
- ☐ Camera or video camera
- ☐ Phone or e-mail list of those to inform when baby arrives
- ☐ Journal to record your thoughts
- ☐ Books or magazines to pass the time
- ☐ Music

Prayer Concerns

Baby's final stages of development
Mommy's comfort
Labor and delivery
A healthy baby!

A Prayer for Labor and Delivery

Dear Lord,

Thank you for being with me through these past forty weeks. Your amazing grace has helped me through every moment. I ask you to keep your hand on my sweet child during the birth process. Please keep baby's heart strong and help the doctors and nurses know exactly what to do in every possible situation. I trust you, Lord, to be with us both so that after this short time of pain and discomfort, I will finally and joyfully hold this precious life in my arms. Amen.

Write a prayer here for your own personal journey.

_____

_____

_____

_____

_____

Journal

Record your thoughts and your fears here. It is important to acknowledge every thought and feeling you are experiencing. The main thing is to get them out in the open, and if they do not line up with the truth or the faith that you possess, then get rid of those burdens by giving them over to your Pregnancy Companion.

_____

_____

_____

_____

_____

Chapter Ten

Fighting Fear
High-Risk Pregnancies, Complications, and Loss

Key Bible Verses

*Therefore we do not lose heart. Though outwardly we are wasting
away, yet inwardly we are being renewed day by day. For our light and
momentary troubles are achieving for us an eternal glory that far outweighs them all. So we fix our eyes not on what is seen, but on what is
unseen. For what is seen is temporary, but what is unseen is eternal.*
2 Corinthians 4:16–18

Let us hold unswervingly to the hope we profess, for he who promised is faithful.
Hebrews 10:23

For most of you, this chapter will be completely unnecessary. For others, it will
be a source of curiosity or a double check to make sure things are OK. For a
small minority, this chapter will be a resource if your pregnancy falls in the high-
risk category. When the unexpected happens in pregnancy it can be unnerving,
and we often look for reasons to blame ourselves. Most pregnancy complications
are not caused by our own actions but rather by chance or genetics.

Placenta Previa

At your twenty-week ultrasound, one of the things that will be evaluated is the
position of your placenta. *Placenta previa* is when the placenta is attached in the
lower part of your uterus and covers your cervix. A *marginal* or *partial* previa
is where the placenta only covers part of the cervix. This condition will often
resolve before delivery. In a complete previa, the placenta covers the entire cervix,

remaining there for the rest of pregnancy. Placenta previa is very rare, occurring in .25 percent of pregnancies.

The placenta is full of blood vessels that help to bring nutrition to the baby. If the placenta is over the cervix and the cervix opens, this can cause the blood vessels to be disturbed and serious bleeding to occur. So if you have placenta previa and have any bleeding at all, you will be instructed to go to the hospital right away.

Placenta Previa

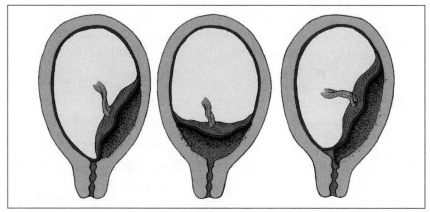

© 2010 Wolters Kluwer Health | Lippincott Williams and Wilkins

With placenta previa, you must avoid any activity that might put pressure on the cervix. This includes sex and cervical examinations. Your doctor may or may not limit your exercise. If you do have bleeding, you may need to be on bed rest. If the bleeding is heavy, then the doctor will deliver the baby. If you have placenta previa, then you will need a cesarean section.

Things that increase your chances of having placenta previa are:

- Age greater than thirty-five
- Having more than five children
- Smoking
- Previous cesarean delivery

Placenta previa is a rare but serious complication. Great advances have been made with ultrasound, so we can know in advance the placenta's location and take every precaution to prevent excessive bleeding.

Preeclampsia

Preeclampsia is elevated blood pressure (greater than 140/90) and evidence of poorly functioning kidneys (protein in your urine) that occurs after twenty weeks of pregnancy. It may have other symptoms like headache, swelling, and upper abdominal pain. Preeclampsia can cause severe complications such as stroke, stillbirth, and seizure (which is called *eclampsia*).

Yes, that all sounds a little scary, but the good news is that with careful monitoring, doctors can usually intervene before the syndrome becomes severe.

Many moms will have slightly elevated blood pressure during pregnancy. If this happens, your doctor will most likely do extra tests to make sure that you are not developing preeclampsia. Additionally, you may be placed on bed rest and required to make extra visits to the hospital for blood pressure checks. One lovely test you might get to do, if you're lucky, is a 24-hour urine test. This involves collecting your pee for an entire day and bringing it to the office. Yes, when you have elevated blood pressure, we are often not content with the little cup sample you give us—we need more of it to study your kidney functions.

When the blood pressure and urine tests begin to show signs of worsening or if the health of you or the baby is uncertain, then your doctor will most likely proceed with delivery. You can often have a vaginal delivery, but if the baby begins to show signs of distress, a cesarean section is likely.

Things that increase your risk of preeclampsia:

- This is your first pregnancy
- Chronic hypertension
- Diabetes
- Obesity
- Twins
- Age greater than thirty-five

Preterm Labor

Preterm labor is defined as contractions that cause cervical change before thirty-seven weeks. This can be extremely stressful and confusing because the majority of pregnant women will experience symptoms of preterm labor at some point in their pregnancy, but only about eleven percent will actually deliver early. The incidence of delivery before thirty-two weeks is even lower, at two percent of total births in the U.S. It is these extremely early deliveries that are most associated with the long-term complications of premature delivery such as cerebral palsy and vision problems.

Symptoms

The most common symptom of preterm labor is contractions. However, a lot of women will have contractions from time to time. If you experience more than six contractions in an hour, then drink several large glasses of water and rest. The hormone that tells your body that you are dehydrated is very similar in shape to the hormone that tells your uterus to contract. If you continue to have more than six contractions in an hour, then notify your doctor.

Vaginal bleeding can be another sign of preterm labor. Any vaginal bleeding in pregnancy should be evaluated immediately. The evaluation will usually include an ultrasound to look at the placenta and an evaluation of the cervix. Often the bleeding is coming from the cervix itself and is nothing to worry about; however, it could be a sign of preterm labor or placenta previa, which can be very serious.

Other symptoms of preterm labor are back pain, pelvic pressure, and watery discharge. These symptoms are common in healthy pregnant women as well, so the key is to seek medical attention if these symptoms are a change for you. If you suddenly feel a constant pressure like you need to have a bowel movement (and you don't) then this should be evaluated. A severe back pain that is new should also be evaluated. A watery discharge that continues to come out even after fully emptying your bladder could be a sign of your water breaking, so this should also prompt a visit to your doctor.

Preterm labor symptoms include:

- Contractions (more than six in an hour)
- Pelvic pressure
- Vaginal bleeding
- Low back pain
- Watery vaginal discharge

Risk Factors

If so many women have symptoms of preterm labor, is there a way to know if you are going to be high risk? There are some risk factors that can be looked at initially, but not all women with preterm delivery will have risk factors. The best thing to look at is your history in previous pregnancies. Yes, I know that's not helpful while you're carrying baby number one.

If in your first pregnancy you delivered at term (after thirty-seven weeks), then this alone means that you have a ninety-five percent chance of delivering at term again, as long as you haven't taken up smoking crack since your last pregnancy. So essentially, your first pregnancy is the litmus test for how your cervix will behave.

Things that increase your risk of preterm labor are:

- Smoking
- Low weight gain
- Illicit drug use
- Infection (UTIs)
- Periodontal disease
- Cone cervical biopsies
- Genetics
- Twins

Some of these things are modifiable and some of them aren't. Getting good nutrition with adequate calorie intake is important as well as taking good care of your teeth. Stopping smoking and drug use is of the highest priority and has the largest impact on decreasing the risk of preterm delivery. We are not sure of the extent to which genetics plays a part, but we do tend to see a slightly increased risk of preterm labor if your mother had a history of it.

A cone biopsy or LEEP procedure is performed to remove an area of your cervix that contains precancerous cells. Having had one LEEP procedure can slightly increase your risk of delivering early, but having had more than one LEEP procedure makes your risk higher. If you have had multiple LEEP procedures, then your doctor may consider monitoring your cervix with ultrasounds.

Recurrent UTIs can also be associated with preterm labor, which is one of the reasons a urine sample is checked when you come for each visit.

Diagnosis

The initial way to test for preterm labor is to evaluate your cervix. This can be done as a combination of your doctor checking to see if you are dilated and an ultrasound that measures the thickness of your cervix. Also, your doctor can put you on a monitor that measures how often you are contracting. The cervix should be more than twenty-five millimeters thick.

Additionally, the doctor can do a test called a *fetal fibronectin* (fFN). This test is a vaginal swab that checks for a specific protein released by the amniotic membranes as the uterus readies itself for labor. The test can be done between twenty-four and thirty-four weeks. If the fFN is negative and the cervix is a normal length and closed, then there is a ninety-nine percent chance that you will not deliver in the next two weeks. So if all these tests are negative, you can be reassured that the symptoms you are having are just symptoms and not preterm labor. The doctor will also give you instructions as to when to notify her if the symptoms recur.

What if the tests are positive? If the tests are positive, it does not mean that you are getting ready to deliver soon, but it does mean that there is a slightly increased risk of delivery before thirty-seven weeks.

Treatment

If you do go into preterm labor and your cervix begins to dilate before thirty-four weeks, then your doctor will most likely give you medications to try to stop the labor if there is no sign of infection. If there are signs of infection in the uterus, then it is safer to go ahead and let the baby deliver.

The main goal of stopping your labor is to give you steroid shots that will help mature the baby's lungs. You will be in the hospital for several days, sometimes for the remainder of your pregnancy. If you are discharged home, you will usually be on bed rest.

Babies who are born after thirty-two weeks will usually have to stay in the NICU for several weeks, but they will generally not have any long-term problems associated with being born premature. If the baby is born at less than twenty-six weeks, then the long-term outcome is not as optimistic. Luckily, this makes up a very small number of preterm births.

Recurrence

So, what if you did have preterm labor in your first pregnancy? If you delivered before thirty-seven weeks in a previous pregnancy, then your doctor will most likely monitor you more closely. Your risk of delivering early is about fifteen percent. One newer intervention for moms with a history of preterm labor is progesterone injections. These can be given weekly from sixteen to thirty-six weeks and decrease your risk of preterm delivery by about forty percent. Your doctor may also perform the fFN and cervical length tests at regular intervals to help monitor your risks. If you show signs of preterm labor, she may put you on bed rest or give you steroid injections to help mature the baby's lungs.

Twins

One of my absolute favorite things to do as an OB is to tell women that they are having twins. The reactions can be truly hilarious. One specific incident involved a couple who did not speak English. As I showed them the two distinct heartbeats on the ultrasound machine, there was no language barrier as I interpreted their reaction. You could see their expressions go from incredulity, to fear, to tears of joy all in a brief moment.

The rate of twins in the U.S. is about one percent of pregnancies. This number is increasing significantly due to fertility treatments. Also, the rate of twins is higher in African American women than in Caucasian or Hispanic women.

Things that increase your chances of having twins:

- Age greater than thirty-five
- Having more than four children
- Genetics (of the mother's side)
- Fertility treatments

If you are pregnant with twins, you have an increased rate of several complications, including preterm labor, gestational diabetes, cesarean delivery and preeclampsia. Additionally, the doctor will be doing regular ultrasounds to make sure that each baby is growing equally. Especially with identical twins who share the same placenta, there is a tendency for one twin to steal blood flow and nutrition from the other. If this happens, the doctor may need to deliver the babies early to help get more nutrition to the smaller one. While they are at increased risk of pregnancy complications, twins can often deliver vaginally at term without problem.

Stillbirth

Stillbirth is perhaps the biggest fear of all pregnant women. Stillbirth is defined as the death of a baby after twenty weeks or 500 grams. The current rate of stillbirth in the U.S. is approximately 1 per 1,000 births. The risk of stillbirth has decreased significantly over the last several decades with advances in treatment of maternal disease. Diabetes, preeclampsia, and Rh sensitization were a major cause of stillbirth only half a century ago. With current prenatal care, we now can screen for, treat, and intervene with these conditions before they lead to such significant consequences.

Causes of stillbirth:

- Chromosomal abnormality
- Infections
- Abruption
- Cord accident
- Trauma
- Postterm pregnancy
- Drug use
- Unknown

One thing you can do is to make sure you always wear your seat belt. Women often worry about the lap belt hurting their uterus, but the risk of trauma without seat belts is much higher. If you are involved in any sort of trauma, even if you do not directly hurt your belly, you should seek medical attention immediately.

An umbilical cord accident is another thing that moms often worry about. The truth is that twenty percent of babies are born with the cord around their neck, so this in and of itself is not likely to cause stillbirth. In some instances, the baby can get overly tangled in his cord, and this can result in him cutting off his own blood supply. Moms will often report a decrease in fetal movement when this happens. This is the reason we recommend performing kick counts every day starting at twenty-seven weeks. Remember: movements six times an hour at least once a day.

That being said, there are some causes that are not preventable, such as chromosomal abnormality and infection.

An especially challenging situation is when mom is pregnant, and she knows someone who experiences a loss. It's hard not to think "What if it happened to me?" These are normal feelings. Remember that the overall risk is low. By going to your prenatal visits, wearing your seat belt, and doing your kick counts, you are doing all the right things to keep your baby healthy.

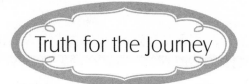
Truth for the Journey

*Therefore we do not lose heart. Though outwardly we are wasting
away, yet inwardly we are being renewed day by day. For our light
and momentary troubles are achieving for us an eternal glory that far
outweighs them all. So we fix our eyes not on what is seen, but on what
is unseen. For what is seen is temporary, but what is unseen is eternal.*
2 Corinthians 4:16–18

Let us hold unswervingly to the hope we profess, for he who promised is faithful.
Hebrews 10:23

Yes, there are two key Bible verses for this chapter. I'm not trying to overload you with scripture to memorize. All right, maybe I am. There are so many wonderful verses that can be encouraging in tough times. As we journey through the valleys of our lives, the Word of God will be our comfort and our guide if we let it. I encourage you to allow the depth of God's love to come and cover you right now.

As I'm sure you've gathered from the rest of this book, I have had my share of complications in conception and pregnancy, and I am definitely considered "high risk." If you are reading this chapter, you may have experienced some type of complication yourself. I suppose we can consider ourselves connected in that way. My pastor once told me that even though they say you have to walk a mile in someone's shoes to understand what she is going through, he doesn't believe that it's possible to fully comprehend someone else's pain. Your response to a traumatic event is affected by your unique circumstances, background, personality, and even your DNA. So although I could never fully understand exactly what you are going through, I hope and pray that this book offers you some level of peace as you walk out your own journey. Be honest with yourself and God and even your family and friends about the difficulty you are facing.

The two key Bible verses for this chapter are very important in understanding and accepting the story God is writing for you as you pursue motherhood. Each one addresses a different aspect of faith during difficult times. Because I believe that all things work together for our good and the good of the kingdom of God, I hope to help you look beyond the immediate trial you are experiencing.

In 2 Corinthians, Paul is speaking from a place of crisis within the church. Despite their tensions, he is encouraging the church to look beyond their circumstances to eternity. I know the last thing you want to think about right now is eternity, believe me. Especially if you've lost a baby and all you can imagine is that little one in heaven instead of your arms. The truth is, though, that God has plans for every life that reach way beyond this earth. We absolutely have to keep an eternal perspective on things if we are going to make sense out of any of it.

I believe that life begins at conception, so I know that the four babies I have lost in my womb are now in heaven. I've convinced myself that God has an army of worshipping babies that never graced this earth and that their worship is as sweet as honey to our Lord. Now don't think I'm trying to promote my views of heaven as gospel. I actually have no idea what heaven will be like. I know it will be wonderful, and I hope when I get there, I'll be able to meet those precious souls that I lost here on earth. But this small baby-worship scenario is just something I imagine that has helped heal my heart. My point is, we can try to make sense of our light and momentary trouble by fixing our eyes on what is unseen and eternal.

Paul also talks about our trials achieving for us an eternal glory, which far outweighs them all. One of the most powerful testimonies of a person walking through difficulty is his or her response to it. People are watching all around you. Believers and nonbelievers alike want to see how you respond to your situation. Will you react with deep faith, or will you stumble under the weight of your reality? One of the greatest ways we can bring glory to God is through our response to circumstance.

Let us hold unswervingly to the hope we profess, for he who promised is faithful. Do you believe that? It is more than all right to be honest with God about how you are feeling. It is completely normal to have hard days and sad days as you walk through a difficulty like this. He knew you were going to walk through this valley long before you approached it, and he is ready to walk by your side to the very end. And because of that great love and companionship, at the end of the day we should be able to stand up and confess that he is good, because it's true.

Letting Go

If you have experienced loss through miscarriage or stillbirth, no words that I write here are going to take away your grief. Were there words that I knew would take away your pain, I would beg the Lord to give them to me now. But nothing will bring you true peace and resolution besides his mercy and love. Perhaps the best thing you can do for your heart right now is to put down this book. Let go of the idea of pregnancy and babies until you are ready again. God will show you when it's time. Meanwhile, focus on the healing of your heart. I can remember feeling a rush of strength eventually after each of my losses. It was as if the experiences, once faded, made me feel like a stronger woman of God. Likewise, I pray that this process, although terribly hard and painful, will ultimately deepen your relationship with him.

Prayer Concerns

Complications in pregnancy

Dealing with pregnancy loss

Faith to believe for a healthy baby

A Prayer of Declaration

After our first two miscarriages, we felt we needed a strong prayer of declaration to keep our mind focused as we believed for a child. During my third pregnancy, we prayed this prayer daily. No matter what your personal outcome, pray this prayer with great faith that God can and will respond according to his will.

Dear Lord,

I declare that you are the author and giver of life. Your Word says that all things have been created through you and for you. You are before all things, and in you all things hold together. Today I ask that the spirit of life be on me and in me, providing everything that this baby and my body need to bring forth life to the glory of God. I stand on the goodness and faithfulness of you, Lord, that will bless us with this healthy and whole child. May my life and his bring glory and honor to you. In Jesus' name, Amen.

Write a prayer here for your own personal journey.

_____

_____

_____

_____

_____

Journal

Record your thoughts and your fears here. It is important to acknowledge every thought and feeling you are experiencing. The main thing is to get them out in the open, and if they do not line up with the truth or the faith that you possess, then get rid of those burdens by giving them over to your Pregnancy Companion.

_____

_____

_____

_____

_____

Chapter Eleven

Does This Thing Come with a Manual?

Postpartum Care

Key Bible Verse

Lo, children are an heritage of the Lord: and the fruit of the womb is his reward.

Psalms 127:3 KJV

But the wisdom that comes from heaven is first of all pure; then peace-loving, considerate, submissive, full of mercy and good fruit, impartial and sincere.

James 3:17

Now the fun really begins!

Physical Changes

There are a lot of crazy things going on in your body in the first weeks after delivery. All the adaptations that your body had to make over the last forty weeks now have to be reversed in a matter of days. With the delivery of the baby and the placenta, there is an automatic change in hormones. Additionally, you will probably feel very emotional over the next few weeks. This is caused by a combination of hormones and sleep deprivation.

Your body requires fifty percent more blood and fluid during pregnancy. Some of this fluid is lost as blood during delivery. The rest your body will excrete in the form of urine over the next week. So you will be peeing a lot more than normal during this time. You might experience an increase in swelling over the first postpartum week, which may cause you alarm. Moms think, "Hey, I'm not pregnant anymore. Why am I still swelling?" This is often just your body trying to figure out what to do with all the extra fluid that it has floating around. As long as your blood pressure is normal and the swelling is symmetric, this is usually a normal post-pregnancy occurrence. However, if you have swelling and tenderness in one leg but not the other, it could be the sign of a blood clot, and you should notify your doctor.

Your uterus is a giant muscle that grew one hundred times bigger than normal during your pregnancy. It has to shrink back down to its normal size over the next few weeks. Don't be alarmed if you still "look pregnant" over the next couple of days. The hormones released with nursing cause your uterus to contract and help it shrink down, so you might notice cramping and bleeding while breast-feeding. While you are in the hospital, the nurses will massage your uterus to help it shrink. This can sometimes be painful.

Your uterus also needs to shed all the extra lining that was supporting the pregnancy, so you're getting ready to have one long period. Bleeding after delivery can last from two to eight weeks. It is usually like a heavy period for the first few days, then it decreases. At about two weeks postpartum, it will often increase again. The discharge will then feel like a heavy period for a few days, as the site where the placenta was attached begins to shed off. Occasionally you will pass small clots, about the size of a quarter, and this is normal. After you're home, if you begin bleeding heavily (soaking more than one pad in an hour) for a couple hours in a row, then you should call your doctor.

You can now take anti-inflammatory medications such as ibuprofen (Advil or Motrin) and naproxen (Aleve). Although not safe in pregnancy, these are safe for breastfeeding. They can help significantly with the cramping pains after delivery.

The amount of physical discomfort you will experience after delivery varies depending on whether you had an episiotomy or tear. Severe tears are rare and affect less than two percent of deliveries. Even with no tear at all, you are likely to experience some aching, swelling, and discomfort in the vaginal area. (If you don't tear, be careful not to brag too much or your friends will hate you.) Ice packs are readily available at the hospital, and you should use them as much as possible in the first twenty-four hours after delivery.

After delivery, you will be given a squirt bottle to rinse off with instead of using toilet paper after using the bathroom. This will be more comfortable as the skin heals. When patients do have a tear or an episiotomy, they usually heal remarkably quickly. During the first week or so, the area can be quite tender, so after the swelling resolves with ice, you can use a sitz bath to alleviate any further discomfort. A sitz bath is a warm water basin that you can sit in to soothe your sore bottom.

A stool softener can also be helpful to prevent constipation. Your first few bowel movements will be a little painful, though usually not as bad as people think they will be. As you deliver, the vaginal skin will often stretch and "crack" open. These raw areas cause stinging and burning when you urinate for the first few days. You may need to take pain medicine for the vaginal discomfort. If the vaginal pain lasts longer than three weeks, you should notify your doctor. The stitches used to repair tears and episiotomies will dissolve over the next couple of weeks, so you don't need to worry about having those removed.

As soon as the vaginal pain resolves, you can start back on your Kegel exercises. They will help build back up those muscles that were stretched out with delivery. It is normal to experience some leaking of urine when you cough or sneeze shortly after delivery. If these symptoms persist longer than three months, notify your doctor.

During your time in the hospital, try to get as much rest as possible. I realize this can be challenging, but you may need to limit visitors or send the baby to the nursery for a few hours to catch up on a little sleep before you go home. If possible, request that gifts be sent to your house instead of the delivery room. It's stressful going home from the hospital; the less stuff you have to pack up, the better.

Cesarean Section Recovery

The recovery from a C-section is usually more challenging than that from a vaginal delivery. Immediately after the C-section, you will be given pain medicine through an IV pump or through an epidural pump. Often, you will be given a button to push if you need more pain medicine. This gives you a feeling of control and lets you keep the pain from getting too intense. These pumps are set so that you can't take too much.

The amount of pain after a C-section depends on the person and the procedure. If you were in labor for two days, then pushed for three hours before your C-section, you are going to be pretty sore (and tired). Conversely, if your baby was breech and you came in for a scheduled C-section, your pain and fatigue level won't be as high. If you are heavier, there is physically more tissue to heal, and you will often have more discomfort. If you've had multiple cesarean sections and are having a repeat C-section, you may have some increased discomfort from your old scar tissue. The key here is that if you are hurting, *take the pain medicine*.

I will sometimes have moms who refuse or don't take enough pain medicine because they're afraid of its effects on the baby. They obviously don't want to do anything that might harm their little one, but the medicine given is safe for breast-feeding mothers. Having your pain adequately controlled will actually allow you to better bond with your baby. Most moms stay in the hospital three days after a C-section. A longer stay allows you adequate time to begin the healing process as well as be monitored for any post-delivery complications.

You will have a catheter in your bladder and an IV to give you fluids and pain medicine for the first twelve to twenty-four hours after surgery. You mainly rest in bed during this time. On the day after the procedure, you will usually be allowed to eat regular food and switch to pain pills instead of IV pain medicine. The first time you get up to urinate, you will be pretty sore. Having the catheter removed does not feel too pleasant either. During the C-section, your bladder is manipulated quite a bit internally. You may feel a tugging or pulling sensation when you urinate for the first week after delivery.

Your incision may burn, ache, or sting. Occasionally, the incision itself will be numb and the pain will be on the sides of the incision. The numbness can take several months to resolve. As the incision heals, you may also have some itching, which is normal. Watch for redness, thick yellow drainage, or fever, as these could be signs of infection. If you can't see your incision very well due to the shape of your belly, make sure you either look at it in the mirror or have someone look at it every day at home. When you are discharged from the hospital, you will be given a list of restrictions and instructions. Be sure to follow these instructions carefully.

Breastfeeding

Breastfeeding moms will want to start as soon as possible after delivery. Most hospitals have a lactation consultant on staff. Try to take full advantage of her while you are there. Most are also available after delivery, so if you get home and have a question, make sure that you have her number handy.

You may find that despite being so "natural," breastfeeding often doesn't come naturally at first. Sometimes it's hard to not take it personally when the baby doesn't latch on or feed properly. Just remember this is a new experience for both of you. It may seem that the baby is not getting much milk at first, but luckily God made newborns to need very little milk for the first twenty-four hours. Then during the second day of life, babies usually want to feed every couple of hours. The nurses will make sure that he is wetting enough diapers, which is a sign that the baby is getting enough milk. When you go home, they will give you instructions on how many wet and dirty diapers he should have each day, so you can make sure he is getting enough.

If you are planning to breastfeed, I encourage you to have the supplies you need ready at home. Even if you are planning to be a stay-at-home mom, I would recommend having some type of breast pump available when you come home, even if it is only an inexpensive handheld model. If you are planning to go back to work, then you will probably want to invest in a high-quality portable one; however, you may want to rent one first to make sure everything is going smoothly before you invest several hundred dollars. Also, if you qualify for WIC (see callout box in Chapter Three), you may be eligible for a pump and supplies through that program.

Having a breast pump on hand can be helpful if you get a blocked duct or mastitis (breast infection). Occasionally, a baby will (for whatever reason) eat from only one side for a day or two, so having a breast pump handy in these situations can be helpful to relieve the discomfort of engorgement. I also recommend that you keep some frozen peas on hand to use as ice packs to ease the discomfort of engorgement. Lanolin cream can help with nipple soreness and cracking. Apply it after breastfeeding and after bathing. I personally found it to be absolutely magical. You may also want to experiment with different types of breast pads to make you more comfortable.

Attending a breastfeeding class before delivery will help you with breastfeeding strategies and allow you to meet the hospital lactation consultants. Continue to take your prenatal vitamin as long as you are breastfeeding. Staying well hydrated and feeding your baby frequently is key to maintaining an adequate milk supply, so get used to drinking water constantly. Constipation can continue during breastfeeding, so taking a stool softener may also be helpful.

Common Breastfeeding Issues[1]

Problem	Definition	Symptoms	Timing	Treatment
Engorgement	Breasts that are too full of milk	Both breasts painful and swollen Sometimes low-grade temperature < 101°	3–5 days postpartum	Frequent feeding or pumping Using moist, warm heat and gentle massage before feeding Ice packs after feeding
Candida infection	Yeast infection of nipples Sometimes associated with infant thrush	Itching Burning or shooting pains in the nipple during feeding	After breastfeeding established, not usually seen in immediate postpartum period	Topical gentian violet or antifungal cream Prescription antifungal medication
Blocked duct	Blockage of milk in a localized area of one breast	Painful knot No fever or redness	Anytime	Moist heat and massage before nursing
Mastitis	Breast infection	Pain Fever (often > 101°) Redness and heat on breast Body aches and flu-like symptoms	Anytime Usually 10 days after delivery	Continue nursing Antibiotics Acetaminophen (Tylenol) for fever
Breast abscess	Localized infection that has become a pocket of pus	Pain Fever Localized tender mass	Usually occurs after mastitis	Antibiotics Surgical drainage

The benefits of breast milk for your baby's immunity and growth are well known. For some people, breastfeeding comes very easily. For others, it is difficult. For some, it just doesn't work, and their bodies don't produce enough milk. I think one of the most frustrating things about breastfeeding is that you get conflicting advice from friends, moms, and specialists alike. Most books will tell you not to give the baby a bottle for the first six weeks, or you risk nipple confusion. While this may be a good goal, as we will discuss, sometimes it becomes necessary to give a bottle every once in awhile for your own sanity.

Moms who can't breastfeed may feel like their bodies have failed them, or they are inadequate mothers. This is not true. If you don't breastfeed, you aren't any less of a good mother. If you cannot breastfeed or choose not to, there is no medication that safely "dries up your milk." Wear a tight sports bra and ice your breasts if they are uncomfortable. When showering, keep your breasts out of direct contact with the water. Your breasts will be swollen and sore for a few days, but they will slowly soften up and go back to "normal." Although, after having a baby, nothing is truly ever normal again.

The Doctor's POV: Breastfeeding

I enjoyed the special bond I had breastfeeding my son, and knew that it was the best thing for his health, but by the time my son was a month old, I had the lactation consultant on speed dial. We had every problem in the book: Painful engorgement. Sore nipples. Nursing strike. Eventually, he and I figured it out, but it never seemed as easy for me as for a lot of moms I saw.

I had to go back to work when he was eight weeks old, and I continued to pump until he was six months old. The last two months he refused to nurse and would only take a bottle. So I spent a lot of time pumping and feeding for two months. At six months, with a long road trip looming, I made peace with the fact that I wasn't going to make it to my goal of breastfeeding for a year. I discovered that all the time I spent pumping and cleaning my pump could now be spent cuddling my little boy.

The Patient's POV: Breastfeeding

I knew from the start that breastfeeding would be a long shot for me due to a surgery I had several years ago. Although I understood it would be challenging, I wanted to give it my all. I met with a lactation consultant who walked me through some techniques that could help my situation. I was completely prepared with instructions and supplies.

When my daughter arrived, she was very interested in eating but simply couldn't latch on. Eventually, I was able to use a nipple guard to help her. I nursed and pumped as much as possible in the first few weeks, but I never produced enough milk to adequately feed my little girl. I alternated between nursing and formula feeding for a while, knowing that this stage was crucial for her to receive the nutrients that would boost her immune system. After juggling the two methods for two weeks, we decided to move exclusively to formula for simplicity's sake. We knew that was where we were headed anyway.

I have felt guilty from time to time that I was not able to breastfeed long-term. Although you cannot deny that breast milk is best for baby's immunity, my daughter is two years old and has never had an ear infection or been on antibiotics in her life. I am pro-breastfeeding if it works for you. It is definitely the best option for your baby's health. However, formula has come a long way and includes all of the necessary nutrients that your baby needs. Give it your best shot if you feel strongly about breastfeeding, but don't beat yourself up if it doesn't work for you.

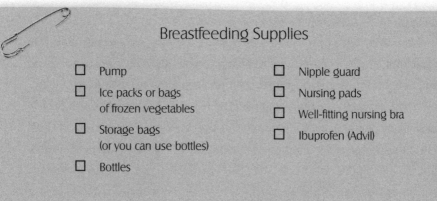

Breastfeeding Supplies

- ☐ Pump
- ☐ Ice packs or bags of frozen vegetables
- ☐ Storage bags (or you can use bottles)
- ☐ Bottles
- ☐ Nipple guard
- ☐ Nursing pads
- ☐ Well-fitting nursing bra
- ☐ Ibuprofen (Advil)

Getting into a Routine

I'm not sure anything can truly prepare you for having a baby. I had my son in the third year of OB/GYN training. I was used to a grueling schedule and minimal sleep. Having literally devoted my life to helping people have babies, I was pretty confident going into the whole birthing process. However, by one week postpartum, I was just as frazzled as all the other first-time moms. I was used to going without sleep on call, but this was a whole new level because I was never off call. The sleep deprivation was overwhelming to me.

Having a C-section, preeclampsia, and breastfeeding difficulties was not the smoothest start to new motherhood. In spite of this, it was also one of the most joyful times in my life. I can remember moments when I should have been sleeping, but instead I would just stare at this beautiful child that had been given to me by God and wonder how it was possible to love another human being this much, so quickly. After a couple of weeks, things begin to fall into a routine, and I learned to accept help when it was offered. I began to relish my new role as mom and wouldn't trade those precious weeks for anything now.

Take advantage of any help that's offered. If your church offers meals for new moms, then take them up on it. If family is able to stay over to help out, then let them. If you are bottle-feeding, let your husband or family member take a shift feeding the baby at night. If you are breastfeeding, your husband can change the baby and then bring him to you to feed, or you can pump a bottle to feed occasionally to help catch you up on sleep. Let housekeeping go, and nap if you can. Avoid as much stress as possible. While some life stressors are unavoidable, try not to plan any other major changes around the time of the birth.

For most of you, there will be a rough couple of days, then you will find your groove and things will be great. My personal opinion is that this stage can be the most difficult for the type A personalities among us: those moms who have read every baby book and figured out their exact parenting strategy before they even reach the third trimester. More often than not, these babies don't seem to have read the same books as their moms. Though the moms do everything they know to do, sometimes they just can't figure things out. When you're faced with a challenge in life or at work before parenthood, you can research, troubleshoot, and usually find a solution. Babies often don't work that way, and this can make you feel like a failure for not being able to fix whatever's wrong. But you are not a failure; you are a new mom! It may be a combination of parenting techniques or advice from your mom that gets you pointed in the right direction, but you will figure out what's best for you and your child.

Depression

What happens if you get past the first few weeks, and you're still having crying spells? While it's normal to feel like a hormonal, sleep-deprived mess for the first week or two, as you begin to get a little more sleep and a little more settled, you should start to feel more like yourself. Even when you are teary and upset, your underlying feeling should be one of joy and happiness as you look at your baby.

Up to seventy percent of women will have postpartum blues. These symptoms are transient and resolve within two weeks. The exact cause of postpartum blues is unknown, but it is thought to be a combination of hormonal changes and sleep deprivation.

Symptoms of postpartum blues:

- Irritability
- Crying spells
- Insomnia
- Mood changes
- Anxiety

If you continue to feel teary and overwhelmed for more than two weeks, or you feel empty or nothing when you look at your child, this is not normal and could be a sign of postpartum depression. If you have any thoughts of wanting to hurt yourself or your baby, or you just want to run away and leave, these are signs of significant postpartum depression. It is important to understand that these feelings are not a result of just your hormones when they last beyond the first couple of weeks.

As Christians, it can be hard to admit we are experiencing depression because we mistakenly view it as a spiritual issue. The truth is, postpartum depression is a serious medical condition and requires treatment. It is essential to treat post-partum depression thoroughly and immediately, so you can fully bond with your baby. I find so many women who want to blame their depression on something: their hormones, their husband, or their circumstances. While these factors may have helped trigger depression, it should be treated as a separate medical condition. It is important to seek medical attention if you believe you are experiencing depression so you can understand your unique needs.

Risk factors for postpartum depression:

- History of depression
- Social stressors
- Diabetes
- Not breastfeeding
- Marital conflict
- Lack of social support
- Unplanned pregnancy

Initial treatment can include social support, rest (sleep), and exercise. Additional treatment can include therapy or mild antidepressant medications. Some moms are very resistant to the idea of medication, but try to put it in perspective. If you had high blood pressure, and diet and exercise didn't improve it, would you take medicine? Hopefully, the answer is yes. Yes, you should pray for healing of the depression and meditate on scriptures to renew your mind, but you should also realize that you may need medication to treat this *medical* condition.

If you do start to take medication, it is usually best to take it for at least a year, or the risk of relapse increases. Since postpartum depression seems to be triggered by the hormonal shifts at delivery, multiple studies have been done that tried to treat the depression with replacement hormones. No specific hormone combination has been found to be effective for treatment.

Symptoms of postpartum depression:

- Loss of appetite
- Loss of energy
- Loss of libido

- Feelings of guilt
- Feelings of emptiness or sadness
- Thoughts of harming self or baby (even if no intent of acting on them)
- Feelings of failure to be a good mother

If any of these symptoms apply to you, please see the Appendix and take a depression screening and give it to your doctor.

Exercise

If you are feeling up to it and are no longer having any pain, then you can usually start exercising at one month postpartum. If you had a C-section, then start with just walking at four weeks and wait until six weeks for more intense exercise. Exercise is especially important if you are beginning to have symptoms of postpartum depression. Women who exercise have lower requirements for medication.

Going Back to Work

If you are planning to return to work, this deadline may loom in front of you. Returning to work is a challenging transition. Just when you have things sort of figured out, it's time to change them up again. Even if you are only going back part-time, it's still going to be a transition. I recommend making a trial run with your day care provider a couple of days before the actual first day back to work. Try getting up and getting the baby there on time while pumping and getting yourself ready. You may not want to leave baby there all day just yet, but going through the motions before the actual first day can be good practice. You may want to figure out where at work you will be able to pump and store your breast milk.

Some moms do great with the transition back to work. I found the first day or two to be fine. (Yeah! Grown-ups to talk to!) But by day three, I missed my baby so much it physically hurt. I had more than one mini-meltdown in the bathrooms around the hospital that week. Luckily, I got some encouragement from other working moms who told me that they had all been there and that it would get better. It did. There will always be moments when you are torn. (Jess and I could write a book about that, too!) But when you are walking in God's will, he will grant you the peace and the grace to make it through the challenging times.

Staying Home

Staying home can be a transition as well. Your reward system goes from extrinsic to intrinsic. You also no longer get downtime. You never get to come home from work. So, even though you are gaining an amazing gift, which is one-on-one time with your child, you may also feel a sense of loss. That is perfectly normal. Depending on how long you were at your previous job, you may lose some relationships and others will change. You may also simply miss the regular schedule that came from working. These feelings are normal and will also get better as you become more confident in your new role as mom.

Expectations for This Visit

Your postpartum visit is usually scheduled for six weeks after delivery. At this visit, your doctor will examine your uterus and make sure everything has healed properly from your delivery. Additionally, she will screen for depression and perhaps discuss birth control options. You should refrain from having sex until after this visit.

As a doctor, I love seeing patients back for their postpartum visit. It is such a joy to see them in their new role as a mom. It can be a little sad, too, because I get accustomed to seeing them on a regular basis. After the postpartum visit, I often don't see them until the next year.

Common Questions You May Have

Will dieting decrease my milk supply?

No, only an extremely low-calorie diet for an extended amount of time will decrease your milk. Do be cautious of going long periods of time without nursing, as this can affect your supply. If your baby begins to sleep longer than six hours at night, you may need to get up and pump so your supply doesn't decrease. Also avoid birth control pills that contain estrogen, as these can decrease your supply.

I seem to be getting conflicting advice on how much activity I should be doing after delivery. What's an appropriate amount of exercise?

There aren't a lot of scientific studies on returning to activity in the postpartum time period. So most medical recommendations are based on medical opinion. Therefore, opinions will be different between different medical providers. If you have a specific area of concern or conflict, then follow the advice of your doctor's office.

When will I get my first period after delivery?

If breastfeeding, you may not get a period until you are finished. If you are not breastfeeding you will usually get a period between six and eight weeks postpartum. It will usually be a heavier flow and longer period than normal. Your periods may also be different than they were before you had a baby.

Help! My hair is falling out. When will it stop?

After delivery (within the first year) it is very common to go through a phase during which you lose a lot of hair. What's actually happening is that all your hair is getting on the same schedule due to the stress and hormones of delivery, so it's all falling out at the same time. It will usually grow back in at a normal rate within a year.

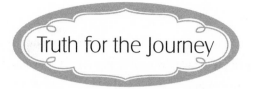
Truth for the Journey

Lo, children are an heritage of the Lord: and the fruit of the womb is his reward.
Psalms 127:3 KJV

But the wisdom that comes from heaven is first of all pure; then peace-loving,
considerate, submissive, full of mercy and good fruit, impartial and sincere.
James 3:17

Congratulations! You made it through delivery. You should feel a great sense of accomplishment. You just brought life into this world! If you thought pregnancy and delivery were hard, now comes the really hard part! One look at that baby's sweet face, though, and I bet you'll decide it's all worth the trouble. I can promise you that life will be different than before, but I can also promise you it will be the greatest ride of your life if you know how to navigate it.

Once again, we have two key verses for this chapter. New parents need all the truth they can get, so I added an extra one in there. James 3:17 is such a great verse because it's so simple, yet so profound. You want wisdom? We're given clear-cut instructions here on how to recognize it. Between dealing with your postpartum body and figuring out what to do with your new bundle of joy, there's a lot going on in and around you right now. The best thing you can do for your baby and yourself is to keep your mind focused on the Lord. He will guide you through this new season.

Your Post-Pregnancy Body

Don't even try to put your skinny jeans on just yet. Unless you are one of those girls who look the same before and after pregnancy, they are not going to fit. Why put yourself through the painful reality of lying on the bed and trying to zip them up while holding your breath until you turn blue? Just keep those puppies tucked away for a few more months. If you can, get yourself a new pair of jeans that fit and make you feel good. It's important to feel good during this postpartum time. And with the right choices and a little diligence, you'll hopefully see your pre-pregnancy body return, and those skinny jeans will look awesome again. In the meantime, try not to focus on the extra ten to twenty pounds you are carrying around. People aren't looking at you now, anyway. They're too distracted by that sweet baby you are carrying.

> There are days or maybe even weeks you live in your sweat pants, no makeup, hair up. If I make an effort to get dressed, put some mascara and lip gloss on, and do my hair, I feel better and beautiful from the inside out. Renee, 21, mother of one

Despite your efforts to rediscover your old body or keep your mind focused elsewhere, you may still get discouraged when you look in the mirror. Try to remember that you are not alone when you find yourself in this place. Almost all women experience these feelings to some degree after having a baby. It is completely normal to feel frustrated that things aren't like they used to be. But I've got news for you girlfriend. Your body is the least of the things that ain't what they used to be. Life as you knew it will never be the same. Your space is no longer your own. Your time is no longer your own. Your body is no longer your own (this is especially true if you are breastfeeding). It's not about you anymore, sister. Get used to it!

Did that make you feel better? I know it's harsh, but I'm actually trying to help you put things in perspective. While personal health and body image are very important, you have just brought a life into this world. You have much more important things to worry about right now. Once you begin to settle into a rhythm with your little one, things will fall into place, and you'll be ready to focus more energy on your body. If it happens sooner, that's wonderful. Just don't beat yourself up if the extra weight accompanies you on this journey a little longer than you would have liked.

Practical Tips for Postpartum Health

- Eat healthy but avoid dieting or obsessing (especially if you are breastfeeding).
- Exercise with your baby. Go for walks with your stroller. If the weather is not permitting, go to the mall and walk with your stroller.
- Remember that it took nine months to put on the extra weight. Give yourself at least nine months to get it off.

Your Post-Pregnancy Heart and Mind

As we set out to create this resource, we asked many women around us what topics should be addressed in a faith-based pregnancy book. Almost unanimously, those polled mentioned postpartum depression. As Dr. Rupe explained earlier, "baby blues" that last beyond the period of transition after delivery is actually a serious medical condition that needs to be addressed. It is completely normal to feel down and not as smitten with your baby for a little while after delivery, but any feelings that linger beyond the first few weeks or deepen into depression should be discussed with your doctor.

Although having a baby is considered one of the most joyous events in a person's life, it comes with many physical and emotional adjustments. If you didn't feel an immediate gush of love when your baby was handed to you, don't feel guilty. Lack of emotion after delivery is very common. You've just completed the most labor-intensive event of your life. If you had a C-section, you've just gone through major surgery. Give yourself a break and remember that love and bonding is built over time. As you spend time holding and gazing at your new baby over the next few weeks, you will be surprised at how your emotions will go wild for your child.

I can remember a few days after my daughter was born, I went into her room at 5 a.m. after hearing her cries in the baby monitor. It was time to get up . . . again. I held her in my arms and turned on a lullaby CD to try to comfort her. She just kept crying. I suppose I thought it best to join in, so I dropped to my knees on the floor in her room and began to sob. My husband walked in a few moments later with a look of concern on his face. "Why are you crying?" he said. "I don't know," I blubbered. "I don't know." The emotions I felt were overwhelming. I wasn't crying happy, joyous tears. I just felt sad. This roller coaster of emotion lasted only a few weeks, and as I began to understand my "new normal," I settled in to life with joy and contentment.

If your roller coaster lasts longer than a few weeks, do not feel guilty, but please seek medical and emotional attention. Talk to your OB and share your experience with a girlfriend or family member. Social support is the first step in meeting your personal needs during this transition, but medical measures may also be needed to get you on track. You should not feel ashamed if you are experiencing true postpartum depression. As Dr. Rupe explained, although postpartum depression may be triggered by hormones and your new circumstances, it is an altogether separate medical condition that needs to be treated as such. Talk to your doctor so that together you can determine your unique needs to eliminate your depression.

Most importantly, seek the Lord for his answers as you navigate through this time. Spending time in prayer and the Word is vital, especially if you are feeling out of balance. Be careful, though, not to make this a solely spiritual matter. While I believe there is a spiritual element to many emotional things we experience, we must also come to terms with what is going on physically. You cannot simply blame Satan or hormones for your depression. Comprehensive care including prayer, the Word of God, medical attention, and social support is the key to getting things in order so you can best enjoy your life as a new mom.

Scriptures of Encouragement

Psalm 121
Remember the Lord your God watches over you. He is your shade, now and forevermore.

Isaiah 26:3 (NKJV)
You will keep him in perfect peace, whose mind is stayed on You, because he trusts in You.

Romans 5:1–5 (Read it in the NIV and *The Message.*)
You can have peace through Jesus Christ because you have access to his grace.

2 Timothy 4:17
The Lord will stand by you just as he stood by Paul to give you strength in order that you might bring glory to him.

Working versus Staying Home

Both Dr. Rupe and I are working moms. We spend thirty or more hours a week (much more for Dr. Rupe, especially when those babies come in the middle of the night) outside of our homes. Because of my experience, I can speak more to working moms, but I will do my best to address the joys and challenges of both situations.

Both working and staying home have their pros and cons. I personally enjoy structure, so spending three days in an office is appealing to me. On the flip side, my job can be very stressful at times, so I am always concerned that it is affecting my ability to be a good mother. It may be hard to think about missing some of your baby's firsts, but there will be many moments you are a part of in these early days. You may be surprised at how sweet your evenings become when you return home after a long day at work to spend time with your baby. Soak up the moments you have with your baby. If you need to work outside the home or simply want to, don't feel guilty about being a working mother. Understand your abilities and your limits and do your best. God's grace will cover the rest.

Practical Tips for Working Moms

Factor special moments into your routine. You may get bogged down just trying to get out the door on a daily basis. Plan time to steal away and visit with your baby, even if it's simply one lunch break per week where you visit him at day care.

Ask your caregiver to send you regular updates on your baby's progress. If your caregiver is a family member or friend, ask him or her to send you picture texts from time to time, so you can see what baby is up to that day.

When you are not at work, don't work. Depending on the nature of your job, this one can be tough. Try your best to leave work at work. When you are with your baby, give him your undivided attention.

If possible, have your baby visit you at work or bring him by on a day off. This is especially helpful when he is a bit older. Let him see you in your environment, so that when you say, "Mommy has to go to work," he understands where you are going.

Try putting even a little bit of your income aside for your child's future (college or wedding savings). Knowing that your hard work is directly contributing to his future happiness may help alleviate some of the guilt.

Ask your spouse for help. He is not bearing the sole weight of providing for your family, so neither should you bear the entire weight of the housework. Find ways for him to pitch in on the weekend or in the evenings after baby is asleep.

If you are a stay-at-home mom, you might absolutely love being with your little one all day long, a part of every moment in his new life. Or perhaps you have a hard time being confined to the house all day. Maybe it drives you crazy that you don't interact with adults on a regular basis. You will likely experience all of these feelings at one time or another. Ask God to show you the unique calling he has on your life as a stay-at-home mom. Pray for perspective to see beyond the routine of daily mom activities. Be open to his leading and be thankful for the precious time you get to spend with your baby.

Practical Tips for Stay-at-Home Moms

Create a routine. Even though you are not bound by a schedule, having a routine will help you feel like you are not just reacting to baby. Schedule set times with different activities throughout the day.

Be strategic. Think about the things you need to get done and set up your baby gear accordingly. For example, create a play area near the laundry room so that baby can play while you do laundry every other morning. Or place his swing in the kitchen so he can watch you make dinner every evening.

Find a local play group. Connecting with other moms weekly is crucial for you. It's also very helpful for baby to interact with other children early on.

Find a hobby. Knitting, sewing, cooking, blogging . . . whatever your passion, find time to do it on a regular basis so that you will feel purpose and accomplishment, aside from feeding and changing diapers.

Schedule your housework in daily tasks. It might seem overwhelming to you to clean your home in one afternoon. Make a list of cleaning tasks and tackle them one at a time during baby's naps.

The decision to work outside the home or be a stay-at-home mom is very personal and is usually affected by personal finances, child care options, and personality. Many women are now striking a wonderful work/family balance by discovering work-at-home opportunities. If you find yourself struggling with the working/staying home decision, perhaps a work-at-home scenario would be right for you. More than anything, it is important to know God's will for your life in this season and to be confident in the place he has you. If he's called you to work outside the home, you will have the strength and strategies you need to do so. If he's called you to stay home with your child, you will find patience and purpose as you seek him.

Practical Parenting

If it hasn't hit you already, now is a good time to come to terms with the fact that you are responsible for another life. Yes, you have a cute little baby to hug and hold . . . but you are also baby's parent! So what exactly does it mean to parent? That might sound like a stupid question. We know what it means to be a parent. We all have them. They've been around our whole lives. We watched ours parent us: How hard could it be, right? I wish it were that simple.

Being a parent and knowing how to parent are two completely different things. Perhaps you have wonderful parents who did a superb job raising you and your siblings. You are sure that because your mom did such a great job with you, she'll just teach you everything she knows as you embark on your own parenting adventure. I can assure you, it doesn't matter how good—or how bad, for that matter—your parents did in their role as your caregiver. You will have to find your own style and your own convictions when it comes to raising your child.

This is not meant to be a book on parenting, so we will not go too far in detail on these subjects. However, we encourage you to dig in deep as you enter your new role, so we've offered a few thoughts to get you started and some advice on where to go next.

> There came a spiritually clarifying moment shortly after the birth of my first child. God would have to bridge the gap between what my child needed and what I could give him. It was too big a job to try to do independently.
> Donna, 56, mother of two

Scheduling

As I write this, my daughter is upstairs sleeping peacefully in her crib. It's 11:05 A.M. and she's been sleeping since about 9:30 A.M. We're going on two hours. I can tell you this wasn't always the case. As hard as I worked at implementing a schedule for our little one, naptime was an issue for several months. It didn't matter what I did;

she would sleep for thirty or maybe forty-five minutes and, like a ticking time bomb, her body would explode with energy and she'd be awake—crying her eyes out. And then, all of a sudden, when I expected to hear her cries through the monitor after she had been down for thirty minutes, there was silence. Forty-five minutes—silence. An hour—still silence. And the naps just kept getting longer and longer.

I know that everyone's personal schedule and preferences are different, so I do not plan to endorse any one method of scheduling. What I want to focus on is the importance of Spirit-led parenting and how it applies even to the practical things like feeding and nap schedules.

Psalm 127:3 says, "Lo, children are an heritage of the Lord: and the fruit of the womb is his reward" (KJV). I believe God desires for children to enhance our lives and thus bring joy and peace into our homes. His plan is for our children to be his reward, not a burden, not an intrusion. To keep this order and peace in our homes, it is important for us to lead the child, not the other way around. I have seen too many families where baby is born and thus begins a whirlwind of confusion and sleepless nights. Of course there is a degree to which this is just the reality of having a newborn, but God has given us access to wisdom and strategy to take the bull by the horns (or the baby by the hand, as it were) and create order for our family.

I read a few different books on scheduling before and after I gave birth to my little girl. I knew the principles I wanted to follow; however, they didn't immediately work like magic for our little one. She was a bit resistant on the nap front, so it took additional time and grace to get her where she is today. Although it wasn't as black and white as I had thought (or as the book had promised), it was so worth the diligence and effort to have a three-month-old that slept twelve hours at night. Your story may be a bit different because, after all, all babies are different. Don't get discouraged if your child takes a bit longer to sleep long stretches or to get on a schedule. Many new moms make sleep scheduling an idol, which can lead to endless frustrations when baby doesn't cooperate. Schedules are not one size fits all.

Breastfeed if you can. Give it your all. But if it doesn't work, move on and don't look back. No amount of guilt will fix it, and your baby will still know you are mommy and love you more than anything! Maggie, 35, mother of two

What If I Hate Breastfeeding?

If you struggle with breastfeeding, you are not alone. For something that is supposed to be so natural, it sure is tough. If you absolutely hate the process of
breastfeeding your baby, I encourage you to tough it out as long as possible. As
you know, breastfeeding is best for your little one, and it is recommended that
you do it for the first year. Give it your best shot for as long as you can.

Think of it like you would any other training or personal health issue. You may not
enjoy working out or eating healthy, but you do it because it's what's best for your
body. The same goes for you now as a mommy. It may seem like a big sacrifice,
but you are doing it for your baby. That being said, when you feel like you simply
can't breastfeed any longer due to pain, lack of milk, your working schedule, or a
variety of other factors, put your boobs back in your bra and don't look back. You
should feel proud for giving it all you've got.

Feeding

Just like scheduling, feeding might look different for each of us based on our
child's habits and personality as well as our own preferences. While we can't do
much to influence our baby's personality, we can help him develop healthy habits
early on. Once again, my goal here is not to push my preferences but rather to
remind you that God desires for us to press into him for direction on all things
related to parenting, including feeding.

I think many parents look at feeding as a casual issue in which they take a reac-
tive approach. The problem with reacting to an infant is that you are reacting to a
brand-new life that is in turn reacting to the shock of the environment around him.
How would you feel if all of a sudden you were pushed out of your warm and cozy
little habitat into a big, cold, loud, and confusing world? You would be scared, confused, and likely in need of a little direction. Keep in mind that for over nine months,
baby has received all of his nutrients directly through the placenta. This whole milk
from a nipple thing is completely new. You may need to show him how it's done!

I encourage you to pray about how you want to approach feeding your baby.
Chances are that if you implement a clear schedule early on, you will be thankful
later when baby is well-adjusted and predictable. Your doctor will direct you on how

much baby should be eating. And baby will need to be eating that much in order to grow at the right pace. Especially if you are breastfeeding, it is hard to know just how much milk your little one is getting. That is why you must be leading the feeding process. Otherwise, your baby might not get the nutrition he needs.

Practical Parenting Plan

Remain a united front with your spouse or support system. You have got to be on the same page if you are going to deal with the issues and decisions that await you. Don't wait until the first situation arises. Begin to talk now about how you want to address important issues.

Get in the Word. Yes, that is my answer for everything. Like I said before, God's addressed it all in there. Take a look again at what the Bible says about parenting.

Be consistent. This is probably the piece of advice we received most as we prepared to welcome our first child. And now I know why. There is no room for inconsistency in parenting. Determine how God would have you lead your child and stick with it. This doesn't mean you have to be perfect. Leave room for grace to cover your imperfection. But diligently seek to be consistent, and your child will respond favorably.

Remember his grace is sufficient. I mentioned this before, but I will mention it again because it is perhaps the most important thing to remember. None of us is perfect. God doesn't expect us to be. Do your best and let him guide you. Just as in all areas of life, he will lead and guide and extend grace when you need it. Thank God for that!

Prayer Concerns

Baby's adjustment to life outside the womb
Mommy's healing after delivery
Wisdom in parenting

A Prayer of Thanksgiving

Dear Lord,

Thank you for this precious new life. I ask you for great wisdom in knowing how to be a good parent to our baby. Help me, God, to know how to lead and guide this little one to thrive in health and happiness. You were faithful to bring this child to us safely, and I know you will be faithful to show us what to do in every situation. We are honored to be entrusted with this miracle. Amen.

Write a prayer here for your own personal journey.

_____

_____

_____

_____

_____

Journal

Record your thoughts and your fears here. It is important to acknowledge every thought and feeling you are experiencing. The main thing is to get them out in the open, and if they do not line up with the truth or the faith that you possess, then get rid of those burdens by giving them over to your Pregnancy Companion.

_____

_____

_____

_____

_____

On Being a Mother

Wisdom is the principal thing;
Therefore get wisdom.
And in all your getting, get understanding.
Proverbs 4:7 NKJV

I've often tried to wrap my head around the reality of motherhood. Well before the moment my daughter arrived, I pondered this phenomenon and likely will throughout my whole mothering life. Motherhood is a gift that comes with a dichotomy of certainty. I am certain I do not deserve this gift, nor can I possibly handle it on my own; at the same time, I am certain that this gift is from God, and through him I have everything I need to thrive as a mother. Some days I cower in fear, believing the former, while other days I stand in confidence, operating in the truth of his promises. The goal, of course, is to believe the truth that you are called and therefore equipped through your relationship with God to steward this precious gift.

I recently saw a commercial for baby shampoo that explained the guidebook for motherhood as, "The perfect combination of the things you've read, your mother's advice, and your own mothering instincts." I'd like to add to that list *God-given discernment*, making our guidebook as believers a complete balance between the wealth of readily available information you can find just about anywhere and the internal personal and spiritual wisdom we have access to through our relationship with God.

Perhaps the most profound revelations I've had on being a mother have come through deep reflection on what it means to be loved by the Father. When I think about his heart toward me and how he responds to me, I am challenged to love my children well. The more I dig into the Word, the more examples I find of how to do so.

The other day as I tried to get my two-year-old to walk up the stairs, she became distracted by every little piece of dirt and fuzz she found on her way (yes, I need to vacuum more often). I was about to lose my patience, when I felt the Lord showing me that this is how I sometimes act when he is trying to get me to move. I look around at every distraction with a heart full of folly. Even though the folly of our heart grieves his, he responds with patience and love, balanced by a gentle kick in the pants from time to time. As mothers, we can much better understand how he sees us as his children, and we can use that understanding to love and guide our own children.

Whether this is your first go at being a mother, or you have a whole brood in your nest, you may experience apprehension and insecurity as you welcome this unique little one into your life. More important than all of the research and studying that you do, more essential than any physical decision you make on how to feed or clothe or diaper your child, your relationship with God is the foundation of your ability to be a good mother. Regular versus organic, breast versus bottle, cloth diapers versus disposable diapers—all those decisions pale in comparison to your decision to put God first in your life and at the center of your family.

I pray that you have felt the presence of your Pregnancy Companion throughout this journey. More importantly, I pray you will continue to feel his company throughout this new season of life. You do not understand the depth of responsibility that comes with being a mother until you are one. Do not let that weight get the best of you, but rather allow it to be the thing that propels you to greater dependence on him.

Remember that God in his great sovereignty chose you to be your baby's mommy. He designed your little one so uniquely to fit into your heart and your home. It may feel from time to time that your baby is an invasion, but in fact he is a perfect fit. His life was created by God and entrusted to you. Every inch of his body, every ounce of his personality, every bit of his heart has been given to you to steward and guide. Lean into God as you seek daily wisdom and strength to guide your life as a mother. You will be amazed at how you will come to know his love for you, his daughter, in a more rich and meaningful way as you fall deeply in love with your own child.

I wrote the words below a few days after we brought our daughter home from the hospital. I can remember feeling so overwhelmed with joy *and* intimidation. *How on earth can I possibly know what she needs?* No matter how close to super mom we think we can be, there is no way we'll get it right every time. Coming to this conclusion helped me relinquish the control I never really had on my little one. You have just accepted the most wonderful, joy-filled, sweet, thankless, unglamorous, and stressful role there is, and you are perfectly prepared for it because of your foundation in Christ. I pray you will accept your limitations early on and let him lead you as he covers both you and your baby through the early days of your life together. Happy Mothering, my friend!

> Ten little fingers and ten little toes
> Oh, how I wish I knew if even one of them were cold
>
> Your little, round tummy I always seek to fill
> Oh, how I wish I knew if you were hungry still
>
> Two bright eyes to see and a pair of ears to hear
> Oh, how I wish I knew the source of every tear
>
> Each and every day I will grow to know you more
> Never really knowing what exactly lies in store
>
> But I will do my very best watching every clue
> Trusting in my God above to show me what to do
>
> Oh, how I wish I knew exactly what you need
> I thank the Lord He covers you while me He gently leads

Appendix

Genetic Conditions That Require Preconceptual Testing

Autosomal Dominant
- Achondroplasia
- Acute intermittent porphyria
- Adult polycystic kidney disease
- BRCA1 and BRCA2 breast cancer
- Ehlers-Danlos syndrome
- Factor V Leiden mutation
- Huntington chorea
- Hypertrophic obstructive cardiomyopathy
- Von Willebrand disease

Autosomal Recessive
- Albinism
- Congenital adrenal hyperplasia
- Cystic fibrosis
- Deafness
- Hemochromatosis
- Sickle cell anemia
- Tay-Sachs disease
- Wilson disease

Multifactorial
- Cleft lip
- Cardiac abnormalities
- Clubfoot
- Omphalocele
- Pyloric stenosis
- Hypospadias

Body Mass Index Table

Body Weight (pounds)

BMI / Height (inches)	Normal						Overweight					Obese										Extreme Obesity														
	19	20	21	22	23	24	25	26	27	28	29	30	31	32	33	34	35	36	37	38	39	40	41	42	43	44	45	46	47	48	49	50	51	52	53	54
58	91	96	100	105	110	115	119	124	129	134	138	143	148	153	158	162	167	172	177	181	186	191	196	201	205	210	215	220	224	229	234	239	244	248	253	258
59	94	99	104	109	114	119	124	128	133	138	143	148	153	158	163	168	173	178	183	188	193	198	203	208	212	217	222	227	232	237	242	247	252	257	262	267
60	97	102	107	112	118	123	128	133	138	143	148	153	158	163	168	174	179	184	189	194	199	204	209	215	220	225	230	235	240	245	250	255	261	266	271	276
61	100	106	111	116	122	127	132	137	143	148	153	158	164	169	174	180	185	190	195	201	206	211	217	222	227	232	238	243	248	254	259	264	269	275	280	285
62	104	109	115	120	126	131	136	142	147	153	158	164	169	175	180	186	191	196	202	207	213	218	224	229	235	240	246	251	256	262	267	273	278	284	289	295
63	107	113	118	124	130	135	141	146	152	158	163	169	175	180	186	191	197	203	208	214	220	225	231	237	242	248	254	259	265	270	276	282	287	293	299	304
64	110	116	122	128	134	140	145	151	157	163	169	174	180	186	192	197	204	209	215	221	227	232	238	244	250	256	262	267	273	279	285	291	296	302	308	314
65	114	120	126	132	138	144	150	156	162	168	174	180	186	192	198	204	210	216	222	228	234	240	246	252	258	264	270	276	282	288	294	300	306	312	318	324
66	118	124	130	136	142	148	155	161	167	173	179	186	192	198	204	210	216	223	229	235	241	247	253	260	266	272	278	284	291	297	303	309	315	322	328	334
67	121	127	134	140	146	153	159	166	172	178	185	191	198	204	211	217	223	230	236	242	249	255	261	268	274	280	287	293	299	306	312	319	325	331	338	344
68	125	131	138	144	151	158	164	171	177	184	190	197	203	210	216	223	230	236	243	249	256	262	269	276	282	289	295	302	308	315	322	328	335	341	348	354
69	128	135	142	149	155	162	169	176	182	189	196	203	209	216	223	230	236	243	250	257	263	270	277	284	291	297	304	311	318	324	331	338	345	351	358	365
70	132	139	146	153	160	167	174	181	188	195	202	209	216	222	229	236	243	250	257	264	271	278	285	292	299	306	313	320	327	334	341	348	355	362	369	376
71	136	143	150	157	165	172	179	186	193	200	208	215	222	229	236	243	250	257	265	272	279	286	293	301	308	315	322	329	338	343	351	358	365	372	379	386
72	140	147	154	162	169	177	184	191	199	206	213	221	228	235	242	250	258	265	272	279	287	294	302	309	316	324	331	338	346	353	361	368	375	383	390	397
73	144	151	159	166	174	182	189	197	204	212	219	227	235	242	250	257	265	272	280	288	295	302	310	318	325	333	340	348	355	363	371	378	386	393	401	408
74	148	155	163	171	179	186	194	202	210	218	225	233	241	249	256	264	272	280	287	295	303	311	319	326	334	342	350	358	365	373	381	389	396	404	412	420
75	152	160	168	176	184	192	200	208	216	224	232	240	248	256	264	272	279	287	295	303	311	319	327	335	343	351	359	367	375	383	391	399	407	415	423	431
76	156	164	172	180	189	197	205	213	221	230	238	246	254	263	271	279	287	295	304	312	320	328	336	344	353	361	369	377	385	394	402	410	418	426	435	443

Source: Adapted from Clinical Guidelines on the Identification, Evaluation, and Treatment of Overweight and Obesity in Adults: The Evidence Report.

Sample Birth Plan

Wolstenholm Birth Plan

Baby: Caroline Hope Wolstenholm (Hope)
Parents: David and Jessica Wolstenholm
Obstetrician: Dr. Heather Rupe

This is a list of my wishes. I completely trust Dr. Rupe and I will yield to her direction at any time during labor and delivery.

Atmosphere

Additional People in Room: Dave (Husband) and Janet (Mom)
Lighting: Low lighting when possible
Music: Option to play music when it won't interfere with doctors/nurses

Intervention

IV: Only if needed
Fetal Monitoring: Yes
Maternal Monitoring: Yes
Induction: Yes, that is the plan
Rupture of Membranes: Yes
Episiotomy: If Dr. Rupe thinks it is necessary
Vacuum/Forceps: Only if Dr. Rupe absolutely thinks it is necessary
Cesarean Delivery: If Dr. Rupe thinks it is necessary

Labor/Delivery

Epidural: Yes, but I would like to labor a bit on my own first so would like epidural a bit later if possible
Positions: Option to move around/walk if possible
Food/Drink: Ice chips

Emergency C-section: Do it if necessary

Umbilical Cord: Dave to cut

Holding the Baby: As soon as possible

First Feeding: As soon as possible, in room, mom to breastfeed if possible (see note below)

Feeding

I had breast surgery 6 years ago. I would like to try breastfeeding as soon as possible but I know it may be a challenge. I am open to doing whatever is needed to nourish baby during those first few hours and days. Preferred formula for supplement: Enfamil Lipil

Instructions from lactation consultant: Feed baby 15-20 minutes on each breast every three hours. Then immediately pump. At subsequent feedings, continue to feed 15-20 minutes on each breast then supplement with pumped milk through syringe.

For pumping: Use Lactina Pump. Set dial to 7. Pump 2 min on minimum, 2 minutes on medium, 10 minutes on maximum.

Supplementation: Take 3 ml of sterilized water and add to pump container to gather all colostrum possible. Insert into 10 cc syringe and feed to baby through syringe.

Postnatal

Baby's Location: In nursery at night except for feedings

Who Will Stay: Husband will stay in room with me

Feeding: Per above notes, I will breastfeed if possible but am open to formula supplement

Pacifier: Yes

Bathing: I would like to be involved with bathing baby

EDINBURGH POSTNATAL DEPRESSION SCALE (EPDS)

The EPDS was developed for screening postpartum women in outpatient, home visiting settings, or at the 6-8 week postpartum examination. The EPDS consists of 10 questions. Responses are scored 0, 1, 2, or 3 according to increased severity of the symptom. Items marked with an asterisk (*) are reverse scored (i.e., 3, 2, 1, and 0). The total score is determined by adding together the scores for each of the 10 items. Validation studies have utilized various threshold scores in determining which women were positive and in need of referral. Cut-off scores ranged from 9 to 13 points. Therefore, to err on safety's side, a woman scoring 9 or more points or indicating any suicidal ideation – that is she scores 1 or higher on question #10 – should be referred immediately for follow-up. Even if a woman scores less than 9, if the clinician feels the client is suffering from depression, an appropriate referral should be made. The EPDS is only a screening tool. It does not diagnose depression – that is done by appropriately licensed health care personnel.

Instructions for Users

1. The mother is asked to underline 1 of 4 possible responses that comes the closest to how she has been feeling the previous 7 days.
2. All 10 items must be completed.
3. Care should be taken to avoid the possibility of the mother discussing her answers with others.
4. The mother should complete the scale herself.

Name: _____   Date: _____

Address: _____   Baby's Age: _____

As you have recently had a baby, we would like to know how you are feeling. Please UNDERLINE the answer which comes closest to how you have felt IN THE PAST 7 DAYS, not just how you feel today.

Here is an example, already completed.
I have felt happy:
Yes, all the time
<u>Yes, most of the time</u>
No, not very often
No, not at all

This would mean: "I have felt happy most of the time" during the past week. Please complete the other questions in the same way.

In the past 7 days:

1. I have been able to laugh and see the funny side of things:
    As much as I always could
    Not quite so much now
    Definitely not so much now
    Not at all

2. I have looked forward with enjoyment to things:
    As much as I ever did
    Rather less than I used to
    Definitely less than I used to
    Hardly at all

*3. I have blamed myself unnecessarily when things went wrong:
    Yes, most of the time
    Yes, some of the time
    Not very often
    No, never

4. I have been anxious or worried for no good reason:
    No, not at all
    Hardly ever
    Yes, sometimes
    Yes, very often

*5. I have felt scared or panicky for no very good reason:
    Yes, quite a lot
    Yes, sometimes
    No, not much
    No, not at all

*6. Things have been getting on top of me:
    Yes, most of the time I haven't been able to cope at all
    Yes, sometimes I haven't been coping as well as usual
    No, most of the time I have coped quite well
    No, have been coping as well as ever

*7. I have been so unhappy that I have had difficulty sleeping:
    Yes, most of the time
    Yes, sometimes
    Not very often
    No, not at all

*8. I have felt sad or miserable:
    Yes, most of the time
    Yes, quite often
    Not very often
    No, not at all

*9. I have been so unhappy that I have been crying:
    es, most of the time
    Yes, quite often
    Only occasionally
    No, never

*10. The thought of harming myself has occurred to me:
    Yes, quite often
    Sometimes
    Hardly ever
    Never

EDINBURGH POSTNATAL DEPRESSION SCALE (EPDS)
J. L. Cox, J.M. Holden, R. Sagovsky
From: British Journal of Psychiatry (1987), 150, 782-786.

Budget Worksheet

Category	Item	Budget	Actual Cost	Category	Item	Budget	Actual Cost
Nursery	Crib			Feeding (Both)	Pacifiers		
	Mattress				Nursing/Support Pillow		
	Changing Table/Dresser			Diapering (Disposable)	Diapers		
	Rocker or Chair				Wipes		
	Bedding			Diapering (Cloth)	Cloth Diapers		
	Room Décor				Diaper Covers		
	Mobile			Diapering (Both)	Changing Pad		
	Hamper				Changing Pad Covers		
	CD Player w/ Music				Garbage Pail		
	Bassinet				Diaper Cream		
	Humidifier				Thermometer		
	Sleep Positioner				Fancy Diaper Pail		
Gear	Car Seat				Diaper Stacker		
	Stroller/Stroller System				Wipe Warmer		
	Diaper Bag			Bathing	Tub and/or Bath Sponge		
	Toys				Towels		
	Bouncy Seat				Wash Cloths		
	Activity Gym				Shampoo/Baby Wash		
	Play Yard				Grooming Kit		
	Monitor				Rubber Ducky		
	Swing				Bath Thermometer		
	Sling or Carrier			Linens	Sheets (Crib & Play Yard)		
	Jogging Stroller				Light Blankets		
	Rain Cover for Stroller				Heavy Blankets		
	Sun Shades for Car				Bibs		
	Crib and/or Car Mirror				Burp Cloths		
	Stroller/Car Seat Toys				Mattress Protector		
	Digital Camera/Video				Sheet Savers		
Feeding (Bottle)	4 oz/9 oz Bottles				Ultimate Crib Sheet		
	Formula (stock)			Clothing	Onesies - Short Sleeve		
	Formula Dispenser				Onesies - Long Sleeve		
	Bottle Brush/Drying Rack				T-shirts		
	Dishwasher Basket				Pants		
	Bottle Sterilizer				Pajamas		
	Bottle Warmer				Sweater		
Feeding (Breast)	Breast Pump				Socks or Booties		
	Bottles				Hats		
	Storage bags				Jacket		
	Nursing Bra				Hangers		
	Nipple Cream				"Going Home" Outfit		
	Nursing Cover				"Going Out" Outfits		

Recommended Resources

Pregnancy Resources

www.babycenter.com
www.pregnancyweekly.com
www.thebump.com
Prayers For The Mother To Be by Angela Thomas
40 Weeks +: The Essential Pregnancy Organizer by Dani Rasmussen and Antionette Perez

Infertility Resources

www.conceiveonline.com
www.resolve.org
The Infertility Companion by Sandra L. Glahn and William Cutrer

Breastfeeding Resources

www.lalecheleague.com
www.ilca.org
www.medela.com
www.bfmed.org
www.aafp.org
The Nursing Mother's Companion by Kathleen Huggins
Breastfeeding Your Baby: Answers to Common Questions by The American Academy of
    Pediatrics

Parenting/Postpartum Resources

www.babycenter.com
www.parents.com
www.parenting.com
Secrets of the Baby Whisperer by Tracy Hogg
Prayers For Mothers Of Newborns by Angela Thomas
The Essential Baby Organizer: Birth to One Year by Dani Rasmussen and Antionette Perez
Tender Mercy for a Mother's Soul by Angela Thomas

Notes

Chapter One

1. Influence of Dietary Fatty Acids on the Pathophysiology of Intrauterine Fetal Growth and Neonatal Development. Consensus Conference: Dietary fat intake during the perinatal period, 11–14 September 2005, Wildbad Kreuth/Germany. Dietary Recommendations for Pregnant Women http://www.early-nutrition.org/perilip/index.html.

2. A. Wilcox, C. Weinberg, and D. Baird, "Caffeinated Beverages and Decreased Fertility," *Lancet* 2 (1988): 1453–1456.

3. Food and Drug Administration and the U.S. Environmental Protection Agency, "What You Need to Know about Mercury in Fish and Shellfish." www.epa.gov/fishadvisories/advice/factsheet.html.

4. Gary Cunningham and Kenneth Leveno, et al., *Williams Obstetrics* (New York: McGraw Hill, 2005), 195.

5. Leon Speroff and Mark Fritz, *Clinical Gynecological Endocrinology and Infertility* (Philadelphia: Lippincott Williams and Wilkins, 2005), 1032–1033.

Chapter Three

1. Gary Cunningham and Kenneth Leveno, et al., *Williams Obstetrics* (New York: McGraw Hill, 2005), 347.

2. Centers for Disease Control and Prevention, "Preliminary FoodNet Data on the Incidence of Infection with Pathogens Transmitted Commonly Through Food—10 States, United States, 2005," http://www.cdc.gov/mmwr/preview/mmwrhtml/mm5514a2.html.

3. Leon Speroff and Mark Fritz, *Clinical Gynecological Endocrinology and Infertility* (Philadelphia: Lippincott Williams and Wilkins, 2005): 1069–1074.

Chapter Six

1. American Academy of Pediatrics, "Circumcision," *Healthy Children* Web site, www.healthy-children.org/English/ages-stages/prenatal/decisions-to-make/pages/Circumcision.aspx.

Chapter Seven

1. Richard Schanler, *Breastfeeding Handbook for Physicians* (D.C.: ACOG, 2006): 37–42.

Chapter Nine

1. Gary Cunningham and Kenneth Leveno, et al., *Williams Obstetrics* (New York: McGraw Hill, 2005), 542.

2. P. Crowley, "Interventions for Preventing or Improving the Outcome of Delivery at or Beyond Term (Cochrane Review)," in *The Cochrane Library* Issue 2 (Chichester, UK: John Wiley & Sons, Ltd., 2004).

Chapter Eleven

1. Richard Schanler, *Breastfeeding Handbook for Physicians* (D.C.: ACOG, 2006).

Index